It's Not About the Food

It's Not About the Food

Personal Stories and Inspiration from Health Coaches and Wellness Experts to Transform Your Weight Loss Mindset and Lose Weight Without a Diet

Edited by *Alegra Loewenstein*

With contributing authors

Alex Brzozowski, Byron Harlan,

Trish Youse Marmo, De'Anna Nunez,

Maggie Paola, Mieu Phan, Cheryll Putt,

Melissa Rosenstock, and *David Sonsara*

Copyright © 2019 Alegra Loewenstein

All rights reserved. No part of this book may be reproduced or modified in any form, including photocopying, recording, or by any information storage and retrieval system, without permission in writing from the publisher.

This publication is designed to provide general information regarding the subject matter covered. Because each person's situation is different, specific advice should always be sought from your medical practitioner. Nothing in this book is meant to be portrayed as medical advice, counseling, or therapy. The contents of this book are for educational purposes only.

Cover Design by: Alyssa Milad

Editor Headshot by: Anna Day

Interior Formatting by: Paul Mavis

ISBN: 9781077049017

Contents

Introduction 1
   Personal Stories & Inspiration 2
   The Pillars of Health 3
   How to Use This Book 5

Part 1: You Are Not Alone 7

Chapter 1: Mindset and Weight Loss 9
   Your Subconscious Loves Metaphors 12
   Wrestling with your subconscious 13
   Find Your Specific Unconscious Formula 14
   Nurture Your Roots 15
   Write Down Your Values 17
   Nurture Yourself in Your Day to Day 18

Chapter 2: You Are Worthy 19
   My Turning Point 19
   Beyond the Surface 20
   Changing My Mind 21
   Changing Negative Thoughts to Positive 22
   Applying This in Your Life 23

Chapter 3: Difficulty Brings Inspiration 27
   My Story, My Trauma 27
   Trauma and Health 31
   Acknowledging The Truth About Trauma 32
   Letting Go of the Old 33

Chapter 4: Self-Care as an Act of Survival 37
   How We Judge Ourselves 38

An Empty Cup 40

How to Fill Your Cup 42

Healing Begins Where The Light Shines Through................... 43

Chapter 5: Low Stress Investing 47

Money Fears and the Stock Market 47

Planning Reduces Stress... 50

The Bigger Picture 52

Part 2: Putting It Together 55

Chapter 6: Emotional Well-Being and Boundaries 57

Physical & Emotional Well-being 58

Boundaries 60

Support 62

Word Choice Matters 64

Chapter 7: Weight Loss Basics 67

Stress 67

Sleep 69

Alcohol 72

Water 72

Happy Chemicals.. 73

Chapter 8: Yoga Awareness for a Balanced Life.................... 77

Watch Yourself Breathe, Change Your Habits 77

Observe Your Body 79

Three Zones in Your Mind and Body.................................... 80

How to Think About Chakras 82

Using the Map in Your Everyday... 84

Chapter 9: Movement as Play 85

An Apple a Day.. 87

    Momentum.. 88
    Outdoors is Best 88
    If It Doesn't Challenge You, It Doesn't Change You 89
    Movement Instead of Antidepressants 90

Chapter 10: Organizing for Health.. 93
    Organizing Basics 95
    Digging Deeper 98
    Seeing Results.. 100

Chapter 11: Food Mindset 103
    Temptation.. 104
    Outside Influence 105
    Emotional Eating.. 106
    Stop Counting 107
    Slowing Down 108
    What to Eat... 108
    How to Eat 110

Action Items.. 113
    Mindset and Weight Loss, *De'Anna Nunez* 113
    You Are Worthy, *Cheryll Putt* 114
    Difficulty Brings Inspiration, *Mieu Phan* 115
    Self Care as an Act of Survival, *Trish Youse Marmo* 116
    Low Stress Investing, *Byron Harlan* 117
    Emotional Well-being and Boundaries, *Melissa Rosenstock*. 118
    Weight Loss Basics, *Alegra Loewenstein*............................. 119
    Yoga for Balance, *David Sonsara* 120
    Movement as Play, *Maggie Paola*.. 121
    Organizing for Health, *Alex Brzozowski* 122

Food Mindset, *Alegra Loewenstein* 123
About the Authors **125**
Acknowledgements **135**

Introduction

By Alegra Loewenstein

I've dedicated most of my adult life to the pursuit of my own health and well-being. I've been successful as a health and wellness professional for nearly five years, and as a science educator for over ten years. When I switched from science education to health coaching, I was sure all I had to do was "teach people the information."

I was very wrong! Within the first year, I departed from the workshops I'd been trained to teach (as part of my coaching certification), and I started creating my own curriculum. (The decade I worked in science education included a lot of curriculum writing, so that was easy!) With my very first client I began to realize that most people didn't simply need information; they needed a process.

I also had an "aha" moment (or smack your head moment, depending on how you look at it). I had personally been victim to knowing a lot about health, yet staying trapped in unhealthy patterns that sabotaged my attempts to "eat better." In fact, it was exactly that obsession with looking to facts and outside sources that actually kept me trapped in the binges, slowly gaining weight, and feeling terrible about myself and my body.

Now I see that I was feeding my tangled emotions. It took me some time to realize that the sugar that made me feel better wasn't nourishing my soul or my body. I eventually figured out how to find the love I so desperately wanted apart from food, which paved the way for a much healthier relationship with food. Now I can eat without restrictions. When I let go of needing love from outside myself, I could then eat all the foods I love, in balance, without overdoing the sweets.

The inspiration for this book came not only from my clients, but from the supportive community of health and wellness professionals – as well as professionals in other fields – that I am blessed to be part of. I receive so much inspiration from the women and men I meet, both in my quest for improving my personal life and also as colleagues. I want to share their knowledge and wisdom, so that you can benefit from this breadth of wisdom I am so lucky to be exposed to, and so that we can all live healthier lives and make a greater impact! (And so you can get sustainable, lasting results!)

Personal Stories & Inspiration

My original plan for this book was to invite this variety of health and wellness professionals to write up their suggestions for best ways you might achieve your personal health goals. Almost every one of the people I contacted ended up sharing the story of their own unique journey. Listening to their stories, I realized that fitness is not about food and exercise; it is about mindset, replacing old beliefs and habits, and developing a healthy self-esteem.

As Trish Youse Marmo put it, "Human beings have been telling stories since the dawn of time. It's how we share lessons, convey important information and pass on our history. It's also how we describe our own catalysts for change, including the decision to break free from the punitive grip of the diet mindset."

So many people who struggle to lose weight are trapped in a cycle of self-loathing or have simply lost themselves in the rest of their life. The idea of "going on a diet" is about deprivation, and to an extent punishment. Until you get to the point when you stand up and declare, "I am worth taking care of," you won't lose weight.

You'll be stuck feeding your soul with pretzels or cookies or ice cream and wondering why it's hard to stop.

Presented here are a number of these stories, from people who ended up as experts in their fields, along with their nuggets of wisdom.

The Pillars of Health

The chapters to follow will bring the perspectives of a variety of wellness and lifestyle professionals, each sharing a story of transformation, along with some essential advice on how to craft a life of balance and joy. As the creator, I reached out through my network to find an expanse of perspectives that would bring forth what I consider to be the pillars of a healthy life.

Flexibility
Future
Food
Freely Given Gifts
Flowers
Fun
Fitness
Free Time
Faith
Friends
Family
Finance

The pillars of a healthy life are broad; I selected these to represent the facets we need to tend to in order to create a life that sparkles! They are not designed to be overhauled in 21 days or 30 days. No one became overweight in that short a time, and no one gets lean in that short a time either. A more realistic goal is to look at your life through the lens of the seasons, over the course of a year, cultivating small steps over time that can be sustained, in order to create big lasting changes.

This book is not a step-by-step or how to guide; rather it is a gathering of wisdom meant to bring about a perspective shift that frees you from the counting and shaming you find in all too many so-called health books. The authors share their journey to inspire you and invite you to take one step in the right direction, knowing that change is made little by little, and it's more important to be pointed in the right direction than it is to taking radical actions.

The pillars of Food and Fitness are always top of mind when it comes to health and weight loss. Of course these deserve the due attention they require when focusing on changes in your health that will result in weight loss. However, most of us spend too much time focusing on measuring these two pillars, so much so that they can actually become a distraction to what is really going on around us.

The personal stories in this book illustrate how even experts have to go beyond the food to make meaningful changes in their lives. In this way, you can expect that the stories in this book touch more on the pillars of Free Time, Fun, Forgiveness, Friends, and Family.

Some of the experts may even surprise you. What does a financial advisor have to do with weight loss? It may not seem a direct link, but the ideas of Finance and Future (i.e. vision, goals, and planning) are pillars of health.

We need financial stability in order to live a life free from stress, which in turn frees us to pursue the quality of life and health we desire. Even if we are living with a high degree of financial wealth, if we are continuously stressed or worried about it, then that wealth is not serving our best interest. And once again, the personal story stands out as the most pressing advice he has to share.

Similarly, organizing may strike you as a non-sequitur in a weight loss book. However, the link between being disorganized and cluttered is strongly correlated with having extra weight. It is common for organizers to find their clients losing weight, and for health coaches to help their clients get organized! In fact, being organized is one facet of mindset that can touch on all the pillars of a healthy, balanced life!

Perhaps the most important pillar of all is that of Flexibility. While being flexible is wonderful for your body and can support a journey to health that will help you reach your ideal natural weight, even more important is being flexible in habit and mind. The chapter on organizing offers support for this essential pillar. When we look at how to organize our life as a whole, we begin to see how to apply a new mindset to every aspect of our life, including health and wellness.

The chapters in this book share both a personal story and a lesson. Getting caught up in specific details and regimented ways of approaching what health must look like is a sure fire way to set yourself up for failure. Looking for ways to connect and be inspired instead will keep you on track for natural weight loss.

How to Use This Book

As you read through this book, remember that the biggest takeaway from these chapters is the change in mindset that I hope you will experience: this might feel like a giant sigh of relief, or a slow, "Ah-ha!"

You will likely be most successful if you choose one small change to focus on first, rather than making a whole list of changes to start tomorrow or next week. Successful weight loss is the easiest hardest thing. More accurately, it is one easiest hardest thing after another.

For example, it can be letting go of feeling fear, guilt, or deprivation, and embracing one small, simple step that you will commit to, for life. Please be aware that lifelong change doesn't mean constantly being strict or forbidding pleasure. . It means developing the habit of making healthy choices most of the time, and allowing for enjoyable exceptions. Every day brings choices, and it's the accumulation of choices that matters, not any single one.

I know that the journey of health is a lifelong commitment. I also know that we all start with one small change. We can't all hire a health coach, a life coach, a trainer, a yoga teacher, a hypnotist, a financial advisor, an organizer, and a therapist to make our lives perfect.

Heck, it would even be hard to read a book by each of these people in a reasonable amount of time! So this book will offer you the wisdom of their stories to provide perspective, as you set off on your path of greater self-love and whole body health. I ask only that you open your heart to be moved, and open your mind to let go of the old ways of doing things in order to take small but important steps towards new ways. The secret to success is small steps that add up over time to big changes.

Part 1: You Are Not Alone

How Others Have Found Their Way to Successful Weight Loss and Greater Well-Being

CHAPTER 1

Mindset and Weight Loss

By De'Anna Nunez

My name is De'Anna, and I am a food lover. I love food the way some people love their emotional therapy dog. I depend on it to make me feel better, to help me access my potential, and to help me address any anxieties or needs.

Okay, that's actually the old me, and perhaps you will relate to how I got there. When I was growing up, my mom did not often share a verbal "I love you" and was not the huggy type. Her love language was food, and she was a skilled baker.

Just about every day after school there were delicious goodies awaiting my arrival home. Some days I would walk in the door to find chocolate chip cookies. On other days it might be lemon bars, or angel food cake… and there was always ice cream in the freezer.

For every boo-boo, I got a brownie. My mom taught me that food was the number one way to sidestep any problem. "Hey let's not think about how awful life feels right now, and go bake some cookies. While we're at it, let's eat the cookie dough, too!"

There were many times, growing up, when I was questioning life or feeling unsure about things. The girls at school were talking behind my back. A boy I liked didn't like me. I got my period.

I missed my dad; seeing him every other weekend just wasn't enough. Mom was not someone I could confide in, and the sex talk never happened. Mom said, "Go read that book on the shelf over there." She was not a hands-on mother in those ways. But what she did do was bake.

Each time I indulged, I felt better – at least for the moment. Sometimes I'd go overboard and eat until my stomach ached. I'd gather all the ingredients for chocolate chip cookies, make the batter, and eat the entire batch of dough before it even had a chance to get to the oven.

Like my mother, I learned that sweets could distract me from what I was feeling; and the taste of my creations would heighten my senses and make me smile, even through disappointment or pain. I would look forward to my next date with a gallon of ice cream in front of the television.

I was unknowingly developing a mental imprint that would stay with me for years. Food replaced the love that I wasn't getting from my mother in other ways. Since she shared this imprint, she didn't mind at all.

Then, in the 1980's, society told me that I should not like myself with the extra weight I was carrying. In junior high, I became very aware of my body with respect to beauty and what it meant to be fashionable. I wanted to look like the girls in Seventeen Magazine. To achieve this, dieting became a thing.

I craved all the sweets I'd grown accustomed to, but at this point, I knew that if I ate them, I'd gain weight and not look the way I wanted to look. My vicious cycle began: Snack. Diet. Snack. Diet. Repeat. Repeat. Repeat. I was on a roller coaster that didn't lead anywhere.

It wasn't until years later, after gaining and losing the same forty pounds over and over, that I went to Hypnotherapy College. We studied the subconscious mind and its mechanisms. It was fascinating to me!

I remember having an AHA! moment: "You mean I don't have to continue to be how I am? I don't have to continue to think how I think?" I honestly had no idea that my mind didn't have to be fixed on my old set of beliefs, especially all the negative ones I carried about myself.

One afternoon, our instructor said, "Please partner up and practice hypnotizing one another. Choose an easy light topic everyone can relate to, like chocolate chip cookies.

Practice age regression and have your partner recall the first time they ate a chocolate chip cookie." That exercise, which was likely planned as an easy and positive experience for most, left me in tears. It was in this practice session that I realized I had been eating chocolate chip cookies to soothe myself, for my entire life.

It was a breakthrough moment! I realized that I had created an unconscious formula: chocolate chip cookies equaled love. In fact, all desserts equaled love. So, every time I went on a diet, that meant to my subconscious that I had stopped loving myself.

How could I stay on a diet and maintain a healthy body weight when my subconscious felt so deprived of love? I need to be loved!

Changing this situation seemed like a monstrous hill to climb, but I'm here to tell you that I did it, and that you can, too – that there is no mountain too big to climb. Come along with me, like a fellow explorer, to see how I liberated myself from the old mindset and found ways to love food and still maintain a healthy, balanced body that I actually enjoy seeing in the mirror.

As we explore for your best new mindset, it is important to be honest with yourself and fearless about what you might discover.

On this journey there is no self-blaming or berating allowed, even as we explore whether you binge, fixate, obsess, coerce or restrict yourself, or whatever other behaviors and patterns emerge.

Your Subconscious Loves Metaphors

Imagine a healthy beautiful body full of energy, as a well-planted flower bush. The green stems that support each flower reach high to the sun as if to say, "I'm confident." We all love that feeling, yes? All of the nutrients the plant needs from sunlight are absorbed by the leaves.

Meanwhile, below the surface, a wondrous root system develops into the soil, drawing all of the nutrients the plant needs from the earth. In our metaphor, what is above the soil is what the outer world sees: appearances and behaviors. What is below ground is the foundational support for what is seen.

When your conscious mind comes up with a health goal, it's focused on the end result, such as, "I want to be lean and have more energy, or lose X amount of weight." You're naming and even visualizing a result.

Most of your focus goes toward tending the flowering green plant sprouting from the soil, not the actual roots of the plant that its growth relies on. They are out of sight, out of mind. Yet, you need to nurture these roots – your subconscious – to have a healthy plant!

Let's think of these roots as the daily habits, conditioned old patterns, and self-image beliefs you currently have and hope to re-direct. Before the plant will flower as you ideally wish, it's important to cultivate and nurture these roots.

Paraphrasing Einstein, "We cannot create a new result with the same line of thinking that created the original." We must show up to the goal with a new mindset. Think of your roots as the path to self-understanding.

Wrestling with your subconscious
When you find yourself eating for reasons other than hunger, know that your subconscious mind has taken over and is in default mode. It's irrational, emotional, and stuck in its ways.

You may say, "I'm not going to eat the nachos!" And then the moment arrives, and you lose your focus. Maybe not every time, because you've been trying to be more conscious... but enough times that you begin to doubt your ability to follow through at all.

In this headspace, it's like you go into a trance. You are experiencing habitual behavior or reacting to some type of unconscious trigger. Food carries deep subconscious connections to feelings of family, gratefulness, love, and more. Using food as a coping mechanism is common, and when we do it repeatedly, we store a behavior in our subconscious mind.

Food is so easy and accessible, no wonder it's a trap! It's also far less shameful than drugs or alcohol. It's one of those semi-acceptable vices, and you can get away with it amongst your family and friends without getting called out. At least, until it becomes obvious that it's a real problem for you, or someone shouts, "Hey Chubby!" (Yea that actually happened to me.)

Some may shop, others gamble, others have sex, but we eat. Somewhere along the way some of us learned that food makes us feel good. Not like, "I feel better now because my hunger is sated," but more like, "I feel better now that I've eaten this food that has magical unicorn powers."

There is an unconscious charge, a spark that happens; to perk us up when we're feeling bored, unhappy, or stressed... or to enhance the joy when we're celebrating. It feels so good! The taste can be so wonderfully inspiring, sometimes we even hang out with it like it's our muse!

We end up using food to make us feel more alive, or to numb us from our current pain. In that moment, it's as if two wires have connected. Bam! Food equals soothing. Your brain got the message that food solved the problem. Now, because we are humans that feed off pleasure, and we'll do anything to stay out of pain or discomfort, food can quickly become our problem solver of choice. We create an unconscious formula.

When I feel _____, I eat _____, and I feel better. Albeit temporary, it does work. Then we repeat, repeat, repeat. Each time we repeat we are creating a defined imprint in the walls of our minds, carving that neural pathway a little deeper. Our subconscious is recording the repetition, and it becomes ingrained.

Find Your Specific Unconscious Formula

It's important to identify your unconscious formula, which usually looks like this:

When I feel _____, I eat _____, and I feel better.

Mine was:
When I feel lonely, I eat chocolate chip cookies, and I feel better.

These days, I call that formula an "untruth", because it once seemed true, but on a deeper level it's not. I did not need food to bring me love. In fact, it's impossible. Food is not responsible for our happiness, self-esteem, or worthiness.

 Food is nutrients and energy! It can heal our bodies with macro and micronutrients, but our emotional wellness is the work of our minds and hearts.

Once I uncovered my formula and realized it was an untruth, I was stunned that, in a sense, I had been lying to myself for all those years. I was shocked that I had been living by a faulty formula, and it was making me fat and unhappy. When we use our subconscious formula to unearth and recognize our untruths, we can then trim them away, making room for fresh new growth.

Take some time to list your unconscious formula. It may be helpful to let your mind wander, or to write in a journal. Ask yourself "What responsibility am I putting on food?" You may even end up with more than one formula.

I invite you to be an explorer of your truth, and explore for the subconscious thoughts that are keeping you trapped. Your truth is the core of self-value inside you. The part of you that says, "I am learning to love myself, and I deserve to actually get my needs met."

Nurture Your Roots

Oprah says, "Once you know, you can't say you don't know." That was true for me, and it is for you, too. You can't hide from the truth once it's revealed. And you don't want to! The truth is beautiful. It can sting for a minute, but it levels the playing field.

Exploring your truth about why you use food in ways other than to fuel your body is exactly the place to start your healing and make good headway. It will provide you a whole new mindset! Being OK with knowing, being fully aware of why you are doing what you are doing, and beginning to learn how to make a new conscious choice, is emotional intelligence.

Your EQ is growing and you're learning how to manage your mind more efficiently. This conscious mindset will enable you to live a more joyous, balanced life.

When you eat for the wrong reasons, you are simply trying to fulfill a void, or a need. But once you compassionately call yourself out, you get to actually meet those needs in more healthful ways! This is when the awesomeness happens. You can learn and grow and discover alternative ways to receive what you need.

This process can be uncomfortable; the old ways kept you safe and sound in your comfort zone, and it feels comfy to be dysfunctional if that's how you've been for years. Straightening ourselves out can feel weird! But the best soil to grow from is the kind that is rich in the truth.

So, what do you do once you know the truth? You grow flowers. And you do that by nurturing your roots.

You start creating habits that align with your new goals. You start being more empathetic towards yourself. You stop beating yourself up when you cheat on a diet, and in fact, you get rid of the word "cheat" altogether. You can journal about difficult moments. You can also make a conscious powerful choice to divert to a new behavior.

Research behavioral scientists have revealed that when you want to break a habit, you can't just stop the habit. You must replace the habit with something else or something better.

So, go for a walk when you're stressed, rather than to happy hour with nachos and a margarita after work. Come up with a list of ten things you can enjoy doing to soothe the specific emotion you had been covering up with food.

Some people say, "I just like food." Or, "I don't feel as satisfied when I eat healthy." If you are one of them, you just haven't made the shift in your mind. Here's one way to do it.

Write Down Your Values

Establishing values and living by them daily can change your life. This incredibly simple assignment will be the beginning of this change: get out a piece of paper and a pen. Light a candle and create a personal ceremonial experience.

Now, place your hand on your heart. This pose has been shown to create a synergetic charge between mind and body. Take four to six deep inhales and exhales, each time relaxing into your body.

Ask yourself, "What do I value most now, based on what I've overcome?"

Write down all the most important ideas that come.

Now ask yourself "Why do I want to live a vital life?"
Write these answers down, too.

Read your list every morning. You can also record the list using voice memo on your phone and then listen to the items as affirmations. I promise they will resonate much more than anything you can read from a book. They are affirmations personal to you!

For example, having overcome the hungry heart syndrome – always looking for love in the refrigerator or the local fro-yo shop – I've learned that real love is all around me. Love is one of my core values.

My mother has passed, and I cannot ever get those years back, nor change her to give me the love I needed from her. But I can respect my needs enough to know that I can extend and receive love with the people who are receptive: my children, my incredible hubby and loving mother-in-law, my amazing friends and clients, even my dog!

I can recognize and appreciate that the Universe has provided for me in ways that are truly meaningful. All I have to do is receive. I found that Love was everywhere when I let down my guard to allow it. And becoming the best, healthiest version of yourself boils down to self-love.

Take the time now to identify your own core values, and remind yourself of them daily. This is how you nurture your roots.

Nurture Yourself in Your Day to Day

Why would anyone want to stunt their own growth? Not you. Not me. At least not intentionally. This is why we must, in developing a growth mindset for healthy weight management, consider the influence of the stored information in the subconscious mind.

Brain imagery conducted through neuroscience shows us that our ability to self-regulate increases our happiness and confidence, and that we all have the ability to grow new neural pathways. Your own brain wants to you evolve! By adopting the insights in this book you can save yourself years of suffering and struggling.

You will also engage in a process that you can start today. Not a year from now once you've lost weight, but now, as a means to incorporate the principles and live them in your daily awareness. It all starts with simply telling yourself, "I can." Because you are meant to be a miracle, and your time is now.

CHAPTER 2

You Are Worthy

By Cheryll Putt

My Turning Point

I was in my mid-twenties when I got my first steady boyfriend. Prior to him, I had only dated one boy in high school for four months. People used to tell me that it was because I was so pretty that boys were intimidated to ask me out. I was convinced that it was because I had no boobs. Essentially, if there was a Zero-A cup, that was me. To top it off, I was shy and had extremely low self-esteem.

One weekend, this boyfriend and I decided to drive to Vegas for some fun. On one night, the plan was to go to a burlesque show with topless dancers. I was mortified, embarrassed, and questioned his motives. But, I admit, I was also curious. Soon after the act began, I was incredulous at all the different bodies that were displayed in front of me. There were breasts of all sizes, and I couldn't believe it!

There were tall women, short women, light women, dark women, thin women, voluptuous women. As I watched, I found myself drawn to a woman who looked much like me. She seemed so proud as she moved around on stage. I told myself that if she could love her body enough to put it out there for everyone to see, then it was possible for me to love myself too.

That was my first profound shift regarding how I felt about myself. I don't know why that one incident moved me so deeply, but it did. Seeing someone who looked like me move with confidence, while a room of eyes focused on her exposed body, was profound. It was a step in a direction that, unfortunately, I would not continue until much later in life. Still, from that point on, I no longer felt ashamed of my body.

Beyond the Surface

What I didn't realize at the time though, was that loving yourself is not just about how you see yourself physically. It is also about how you see yourself personally, professionally, in all your different roles and hats, and most of all, internally.

I had always lived my life for everyone's happiness but my own. I got married, had children, and did the requisite things one is supposed to do. This, of course, is a slippery slope because it is impossible to make everyone happy. As well, when you focus your whole being on this concept, you begin to deflate, lose confidence, and ultimately feel like a failure. You empty yourself.

Hitting the age of 40 was like hitting a wall. I like to call my experience a "midlife revelation" rather than a "midlife crisis."As if a light switch had suddenly turned on, I could see the unhappiness that surrounded me. I realized that my life really wasn't what I wanted it to be. The disappointment caused me to become negative, depressed, and anxious. I had been lying to myself, believing that the things I did for everyone else were enough to keep me happy and fulfilled.

Ironically, with my personality and my training as a therapist, I am adept at noticing how other people hinder themselves from reaching their full potential of a happy, healthy life. But, like pretty much most of us, what I recognize in other people, I ignore in myself.

I didn't know how I'd gotten to this place. I didn't know how I'd slipped into a constant state of unhappiness. All I know is that I started to think, "I'm about to turn 40! I deserve to be loved and cherished! I deserve to be supported and empowered! I deserve enjoyment! I deserve to feel happy in life!"

Feeling worthless, I realized that I needed to make a change for my family's well-being, as well as my own. I searched within myself to figure out my next step. It was time to move in a new direction that would help me finally live the life I wanted.

Changing My Mind

One of the core tenets of my therapy practice and my coaching business is the idea that our beliefs determine our thoughts, which determine our feelings, which in turn determine our actions, which impact our thoughts, and so on.

As I approached 40, I believed that I was worthless. I believed that I was the worst mother, wife, daughter, and friend. While I was actively aware of many of these negative thoughts, most were running silently on autopilot behind the scenes.

I called this collection of critical thoughts my inner bully, and she created more depression and dissatisfaction with my life, which left me unmotivated, hopeless, and irritable all of the time.

Changing your beliefs is not accomplished in one day. You have to be intentional about it. You have to actively and consistently refute your current belief and deliberately create actions in your life that support the new view.

My life-changing journey started on a whim the year I turned 40. I had never before given up anything for Lent, but I felt this could be a good starting point for improvement. I had no clue when Lent began, but a Google answer determined it was the very next day. I chose to give up negative thoughts about myself and others. In the days ahead, I tried to stay mindful.

Changing Negative Thoughts to Positive

The very next morning, I had dropped my children off at school and returned home to shower for work. The water felt so refreshing as the warm meditational pulse of the drops hit my skin.

And then I thought, "I hate that I like this so much. I've got so many things to do, and now I'm just wasting time."

Remembering my plan, my inner dialogue argued that there was nothing wrong with enjoying peace and quiet, that it was OK to say that I loved this moment, and enjoy it a little bit longer. Taking a deep breath, I relaxed and enjoyed a few extra minutes.

From that point on, every chance I had, I would challenge the negative thoughts. I would question my inner bully, shine the bright light in her eyes as I interrogated her statements. Is this thought really true? Is it really an absolute? When have I observed the opposite of this thought? What proof can refute it?

Slowly but surely, I recognized the many negative thoughts that plagued me daily! Our brains are actually wired to look for the negatives. In the early days, before our modern safety and comfort, humans had to constantly be aware of dangers to stay alive. Even though circumstances have changed, our brains are still wired the same. Humans continue to focus on negatives in others and ourselves, instead of the positives. We discourage "tooting your horn" and welcome the opposite, no matter how uncomfortable and unhappy it makes us.

For me, as I began to actively challenge myself, a curious thing happened. Each time I refuted a negative thought and replaced it with a positive more realistic thought, I felt lighter. Each negative thought had been a lead weight keeping me down. As I learned to let go of each one, I lifted a little more. This is the secret to lasting change, both mental and physical.

Over time, I have become adept at challenging my negative thoughts. Sometimes it is exhausting when the bully inside is headstrong. Most of the time, though, challenging negative thoughts has become second nature.

When my car was stolen last year, and other problems resulted, I remember uttering how stupid I was. But the words were empty. Now they had no impact over me. My mindset had been changed, and my life improved with it.

Now I easily move through hurdles that I wouldn't have been able to in the past. When I am frustrated, I can manage my feelings. They no longer take over my whole being, because I have learned to use better coping skills.

I can see light at the end of the proverbial tunnel. My positive mindset illuminates the vision of how I ultimately want my life to be, allowing me to steer towards it. I now have the strength to move forward, no matter how many obstacles pop up in my way.

Applying This in Your Life

So, what does this have to do with you? I am sharing my story so that you can find your strength, too. Perhaps you can relate to the disappointment, frustration, and resentment I had. Often negative feelings trap us in habits of self-sabotage. When our mindset is stuck in victimhood, anger, or depression, it's very hard to make healthy positive life changes.

This desire for a more fulfilling life led me to make scary, but healthy, changes to my life. I filed for divorce. I expected that my life would be almost the same, just without my husband. What I found was that being "single-married" is nothing like being single. My ex, and the father of my two children, was absent in every way. I had no home and no money. Luckily, I did have family, and my kids and I lived with my parents until I could find a job and rent an apartment.

This turning point and experience was also when I realized that I have to learn to accept and receive, and perhaps hardest of all, because my bully had always said otherwise, I have to ask for help. What was initially out of necessity, ultimately contributed to my greater well-being.

Asking and receiving led me to emerge out of my depression. Speaking up for yourself is difficult. However, in order to get your needs met, you need to ask, no matter what your inner bully is commanding you to do. This is an essential step to change your life.

I know you are reading this book because you want to lose weight. My journey out of self loathing, combined with what I've learned in my twenty two years as a therapist and coach, has taught me that there is no quick fix. I know that if you want to change your life, you have to learn to accept that you are important and worthy, and put yourself on your own priority list.

You can't just keep pushing on, hoping one day things will change or that some simple life-hack will solve everything. If you've gone on fad diets or lost weight quickly through extreme deprivation, you know by now that those approaches don't work for the long haul. You have to stop waiting for things to change around you, and you must intentionally take action, to make a change within you.

You have to consciously change your negative thought patterns into positive, realistic ones. You have to move beyond the safety of living a predictable, but unfulfilling life, and take those scary steps. You have to find ways to smile more and laugh more. You have to acknowledge your importance and reach out to get your needs met.

Just as I began to feel lighter, you will too. It's amazing how the power of the mind begins to transform your body. You will gain energy, finding it easier to move and exercise. You will gain a positive attitude, making it easier to choose healthy foods without that voice in the background whispering, "Why bother?"

The most basic change I experienced, and that which I'm urging you to take on for yourself, is to build an internal foundation from which to grow. Focus on yourself; practice a positive mindset; ask for what you need; allow yourself to receive.

If you practice these few things intentionally and consistently, you will begin to feel worthy, uplifted, empowered, confident, and peaceful. This is how you will receive the lasting change you have for so long desired.

CHAPTER 3

Difficulty Brings Inspiration

By Mieu Phan

My Story, My Trauma

I was born into an influential and prosperous family, in Phnom-Penh, Cambodia, in 1974. My father was 29 and my mother was 19. My father's family had built a fortune after having fled from China during the Chinese and Japanese war.

My mother's family came from money, but they'd had a reversal of fortunes, so they were delighted with the arrangement between my parents; though my father and some of his family had little respect for my mother and her family.

My father had a sharp mind for business, and money seemed to follow him wherever he went. He even won the largest lottery in the country! Yet, despite having more than he could ever use, he had a scarcity mindset.

He was frugal and had little trust in anyone outside of the family. He also took whatever he could, without any consideration of fairness to others. He could not know how drastically our life was about to change.

In the 60's, poor economic policies had weakened Cambodia's currency. In the early 70's, the war that engulfed IndoChina spread to our country. Plantations and factories faced wartime destruction of land production facilities, rising operating costs from inflation, and transportation disruption from insurgents.

Commodity production and exports dropped drastically. There was a mass migration of people from the countryside into towns and cities, where food shortages added to the inflation.

Ironically, my family had prospered tremendously from the inflation. One of my father's many businesses dealt with gold bullion and jewelry, and there were profits to be made.

Other members of my father's family were also positioned well during this period. Meanwhile, the sentiment of the general population rose to hostile levels between the haves and have-nots.

In the year following my birth, news from the countryside came into Phnom-Penh and my lavish home about the atrocities committed by Pol Pot and his Khmer Rouge regime.

There were reports that the Khmer Rouge army was going to leave the jungle and head for the city, yet few took this seriously enough to leave the country. Most could not believe that the capital could fall. I had just turned 1 when my little brother was born. Later that year, Pol Pot and the Khmer Rouge entered into Phnom-Penh and overtook it by force.

When this happened, the 2 million inhabitants were led to believe that American forces were on their way to bomb the city, and all inhabitants must evacuate within 4 hours. We were told that we would be allowed to return in 3 days. Believing this, and unaccustomed to life outside the capital, the wealthy simply left the city, carrying very little with them. They assumed that whatever they needed could be bought.

Fortunately, my family met a kind soldier who warned us that tough times were ahead. He advised my parents to carry as much with them as they could. My mother's mother made a baby carrier to carry my baby brother. As we now know, 3 days became 4 years of exile.

Cambodia is a lush country, where the growing season is all year round. Food was plentiful, yet most of the produce did not make it to the people. It was being traded to Vietnam for weapons. The punishment for possession of even a small piece of a forbidden vegetable could be a severe beating.

After leaving the city, we waited in the countryside to be allowed to be returned. Eventually, authorities divided us up into groups: men, women and children, and elderly. The groups were divided to break up families and make it easier to control the people; it also helped with managing the labor for agriculture.

These communities were meant to be permanent. It was designed for a new way of living, so people were "equals." Since people built the communities themselves, the structures were simply sticks, twine, and leaves.

We ended up in a camp where my family's food ration included unhusked rice. At first, my mother would roast the rice and we would eat it, husk and all. It was difficult for us to eat, that way. My mom knew we were supposed to remove the husk but she had no idea how to remove it.

Eventually, someone taught my mother to roast the rice and then rub it to remove the husks.

People would save their ration of cooking fuel for lighting or emergencies and use twigs for cooking, instead. Villagers taught my mother how to extract salt from the burnt wood. It was a lot of work, but then we had a bit of salt. Villagers also taught my mother about the local medicinal plants. They took pity on us city folks who did not know how to utilize such natural resources.

Within the first year of the Khmer Rouge occupation, a virus swept through our camp, killing many of the babies, including my brother. The occupiers had separated the able-bodied men from their families, but shortly after my brother's passing my father was released from his duties and sent back to us.

We were told he had been ill because someone had stolen his blanket. When he arrived, our hut was in need of repair, with a leaky thatched roof and walls that needed reinforcement. My mother and I had one blanket that we shared, and his help was welcome.

Sometime during year two of the occupation, we were given a yellow lentil dessert made of lentils, water, and sugar, perhaps served with coconut milk. It was the first time we had tasted sugar since leaving home, and my father was very excited and ate happily.

By that time, in the camp, I knew what death was, and I was the one who found my father's lifeless body. Death had struck my immediate family twice in this camp. I had not been able to save my brother. I had a strong relationship with my father, and once again I could not save my family member.

By the end of the civil war, my father's large family had all perished, except for one distant cousin. My mother had lost two brothers. It is estimated that 4,000,000 died in this civil war, out of 7,100,000. That's more than half the population.

Trauma and Health

I survived, but for as far back as I can remember, I was not a physically healthy person. In my late teens I developed an ulcer, and while growing up in Ottawa, Canada and later as an adult in Massachusetts, USA, I had colds throughout the winters.

There were emotional scars, too. I would avoid confrontation whenever possible, even when it meant avoiding an elementary school friend who simply offered some honest feedback in an attempt to help me overcome my shyness. I had a hard time identifying what a true friendship was, and trusting that relationships with others could be more than temporary.

In my teens and twenties, I would keep myself busy to escape my negative self-image and to avoid delving into issues from my past. For most of my life I felt unsafe, unable to love myself, and guilty for being alive.

There were times when the pain of living was more powerful than the fear of dying. Even in my marriage of 16 years, I was always prepared for the worst to happen, imagining what might bring about a possible divorce, and how I would cope.

What brought about my journey of healing was a diagnosis of hyperthyroidism, three years ago. My husband I had recently moved to San Diego, and to our friends and neighbors it seemed that we were living the Dream Life: living in a beautiful place, married with 3 children, no money concerns, traveling abroad several times a year... yet, I was having episodes of extreme depression, with feelings of deep despair and helplessness.

I felt like I was living in a mental fog, unable to be present for my children, for my husband, and for myself. I had trouble with memory, and the ability to hold an intellectual conversation. I was at a loss about what to do with my life, feeling useless and alone.

As a mother, I was concerned that if I weren't happy, then how could I teach my children to be happy?

When I was diagnosed with subclinical hyperthyroidism, I spoke with a neighbor-turned-friend, who mentioned her own hyperthyroidism. She had consulted a holistic medical doctor, who had recommended dietary changes that had helped her. I decided to try this approach, too.

After two years of a selective diet, multivitamin supplements, and exercise, my blood test came out negative for hyperthyroidism. At this point, my depression had subsided substantially and my brain fog had cleared, but my lifelong feeling of despair still lurked in the background.

Acknowledging the Truth About Trauma

Fortunately, another neighbor-friend had just graduated from a coaching program. When I asked her what coaching was, she replied: "Coaches support their clients in uncovering their desires, and support them towards achieving their dreams." This sounded wonderful to me.

I wanted to believe that I could do and be whatever I wanted. I wanted my children to believe that the world is their oyster. I wanted them to have the opportunity to explore the world, be independent, be accepting of what they were given, and be grateful for whatever came along. If I became a coach, I could help them… so I joined a coaching program.

Coaches believe that each of us is the expert of our own life. Coaches ask open-ended questions and reflect back the answers to provide new insights. This can help the client identify values, and recognize inaccurate perceptions and limiting beliefs.

During the course of my training, I learned to better understand the role that past trauma was still playing in my life, even underlying what I had thought were simply personality quirks.

Example: I have a need to understand the possible outcome of any action, and become anxious when faced with a new task. Through coaching, I learned that one of the reasons I analyze every angle to best understand how things might end up before taking action, is because otherwise I feel unsafe.

Trauma can create a lot of fear, and my go-to place for fear had been either to run away from it, or to push it way down into my subconscious. Now I have learned to listen to the fear and learn its messages.

Another example: I have a hard time relating to aggression. When someone behaves aggressively, my immediate reaction is to become quiet and "disappear". Through coaching, I learned that past trauma caused me to play it safe and not speak out; now I realize that the cost of this behavior is not being able to work through the issue and correct the situation.

Letting Go of the Old

I learned that the values, beliefs, and perceptions that originated from my childhood trauma developed to protect me. However, these same values, beliefs and perceptions were now limiting the adult I've become in a time of peace.

I learned that the seed of unhappiness is living in a world of right/wrong, fair/unfair, evil/good, should/shouldn't, and other judgments. I realized that the people around me I had judged so harshly in the past for not doing more for themselves, their families, and their communities, were actually doing the best that they could.

I developed much more compassion for other people, and started seeing the world through kinder eyes. Now I can look at myself this way, too.

I learned that if there is someone who makes me uncomfortable, there are lessons to be learned by reflecting on what this says about me.

I learned that trauma alters the values and beliefs that are passed down from generation to generation (intergenerational trauma); and that it's important to do my best not to transmit to my children my own difficulties in trusting others, and in trusting myself to handle difficult situations with others. I don't want to teach my children not to trust themselves.

I learned that it will likely be a lifelong process to free myself from my past of living through a war, and the weakest place a person can come from is victim mode. I learned that I can only be free from my disempowering values, beliefs, and perceptions if I can own them, first.

I learned that escaping important inner work through immersion in a demanding job was not the best solution. I also learned that this is a common escape, familiar to many Americans.

I learned that through a combination of coaching and therapy, I could work through my trauma and even come to see it as a gift.

By starting with the changes to support my physical body, dedicating myself to a holistic approach to healing, and making the food and lifestyle choices I needed to make, I could heal myself of the hyperthyroidism and all the physical ailments that came with it.

From there, I could begin to heal on the emotional level. This journey has turned out to be so much greater than I ever imagined it could be; I hope that my story can help you on your path to greater physical and mental well-being. It is so wonderful to finally claim and experience joy in my life, and I wish this for you, too.

CHAPTER 4

Self-Care as an Act of Survival

By Trish Youse Marmo

I was breathing. Existing. Yes, that much I do recall.

I do not remember what time of year it was, whether the sun was shining, or if the birds, which usually gathered outside my bedroom window, were contentedly chirping on their perches. Now that I think about it, I do not recall much, except the smell of days old pajamas and unwashed hair, the filmy, fetid taste of my own breath, and the heaviness.

Whether it was the heaviness of my heart, or the cumbersome weight of my body on its five-foot-six-inch frame, which housed my battered soul, I cannot be sure, but every fiber of my being ached. It ached in a way that belies my attempts to truly express what I felt at the core of my being.

Not even a year before, I had weighed between twenty-five and thirty pounds more and felt great shame. Shame in a marriage that was struggling. Shame in my shortcomings as a parent. Shame in a body that brought five lives into this world. Shame in a soul unfulfilled. That shame manifested itself in desperation and lack of self-care. I couldn't control the shame, but I could control what I put into my body.

I hadn't meant to lose that much weight, but my choices brought me there: first stress, then undereating, then ulcers, then the inability to eat due to painful erosions in my esophagus. What began on impulse, took on a life of its own, and then shame bought my silence and magnified the ache.

The ache I am describing was not new to me, really. The first time I became aware of its presence was when I was thirteen. Back then the "ache" was more like the feeling I would get when I slept over at a friend's house, in a sleeping bag, on the floor.

Temporary. Fleeting. And totally worth the trade-offs: sleep deprivation, the crash that comes after eating a ton of candy, listening to Rex Smith sing *You Take My Breath Away* on the record player and reading *Tiger Beat*. Wherever the "ache" came from, it went just as quickly as getting up off the floor.

My life up until that moment was not that unusual. I came into the world in the usual way, born to two younger-than-they-should-have-been college students, at a time when the race to the moon was synonymous with progress, freedom of speech cost people their lives, and far-flung nations mourned the loss of John F. Kennedy and the dream of Camelot nearly as much as its loyal subjects.

I was the product of divorce in a time when women like my mother and my grandmother were discovering that they had a voice, and I came of age when being responsible for someone other than yourself was a badge of honor. In my case, that badge of honor made his appearance when I was four-and-a-half-years-old; by the time I was eight, my brother became my responsibility.

How We Judge Ourselves

How I was raised had a profound impact on me. Whatever issue my parents had with one another, I know it had nothing to do with me. They were young, immature, and as different as two people could possibly be.

Whatever disagreements they had in their short, five-year marriage, the one thing they both agreed on was loving my brother and me. Still, I grew up before my time, and as a result of caretaking of my brother, I also became industrious, long-suffering, and prone to self-sacrifice. My internalized mantra became, "It is not that difficult! You are stronger than this! It is not worth complaining about!"

With each imagined rhetoric of my own thoughts, I threw down the gauntlet of my own suppositions and stood my ground — I do have five children after all!

The greater the challenge, the more determined I became.

Putting myself through college? No problem! Relationship challenges with serial cheaters? Easy! Raising five children as a "corporate widow" while my husband was away at the job? Effortless!

Except...

It was... It wasn't... Confronting the truth about the challenges of my life has in itself been one of the most challenging experiences of my entire life!

I took the very parts of myself that I thought made me who I was and fashioned them into a template for existence, while these same aspects were simultaneously threatening to annihilate the very person I was trying to become.

Which is exactly how I created the ability to empty myself of all that I was, while trying desperately to allow the anger and the shock and the pity to fill me up.

It worked for a while. In fact, I got really good at it. What I could not see at the time were that the very things I thought had been holding me together were actually tearing me apart: Busyness, multitasking, perfectionism, to name a few.

If comparison is the thief of joy, then busyness, multitasking and perfectionism are its partners in crime.

What I longed for was contentment and balance, synergy and well-being, peace and joy. Not just the fleeting kind, like the kind that you get while you are on vacation, but the lasting kind.

The kind that sits deep in your bones and percolates up from the center of who you are. The kind that I needed to fill the place where the "ache" had taken up residence inside me.

What I was slowly learning was what Nathaniel Branden summarized when he said, "Of all the judgments we pass in life, none is more important than the judgment we pass on ourselves." It was the internal battleground where I was learning this that eventually brought me to the floor of my darkened room.

An Empty Cup

I knew what I wanted; I just did not know how or where to find it.

Looking back at the woman I was makes me want to drop everything I am doing right now and run to her. She knew so much yet understood so little.

Even now I struggle to recall where the shame came from, and I can't come up with a clear answer. This much I do know: If weighing more made me feel more shame, then weighing less would make me feel less shame. Because, although I could not identify the source of my shame, society had an easy solution for me: Weighing less would fix my problems.

Not marriage counseling. Not learning how to communicate with my children. Not nourishing my body. Not attending to my mind. Not nurturing my spirit or faith. Not learning how to "be." Just weight loss.

I believed, at that time, that my weight told my story. I believed that if my weight was less-than-perfect, then my secrets would not be secrets for much longer.

Perhaps you are reading these words and finding yourself nodding in agreement. Maybe you are wondering how you even got to this point. Or perhaps you already know.

I had spent a lifetime giving to others: my brother, my nursing career, my children, but I knew nothing of the concept of giving to myself. Giving to others was what I knew. It was my identity, just as I was convinced that my weight and my body were part of my identity too. Was it? Is it? What did I know?

I knew that my cup was empty. I knew that I had reached an end point. Whether it was truly an end point or merely a pause on the path of my life's journey, I had not entirely figured out. But I knew that I was done.

I could not take another step further. The "ache," the tiredness, the fatigue, was all too heavy for me to carry. After lying in my bed for hours, days, weeks, months, I began to realize that in addition to feeling relieved of my burden, I began to feel "thirsty."

I am not talking about a thirst that is slaked with the act of drinking water. I am talking about a thirst I had been denying for years. Strength is voluntary, and untethering myself from my burden was a relief. I had been carrying my burden for a long time. It was not that I had suddenly become physically incapable of carrying it any longer. It was that I no longer wanted to. The thirst started with the feeling that a tiny individual drop of water might suffice, and it grew from there. Without water I would die, but where could I go to find water in the middle of the desert?

How to Fill Your Cup

I did not know what the answer was. There was no map for the path I sought. Was my faith the answer? Were the answers to be found beneath my bended knee, head bowed and surrounded by stained glass? Did the answers exist within the walls of my therapist's nicely furnished office, where the jar of Jolly Ranchers sat just within reach?

Were the answers hidden in the piles of dirty laundry, lying in the sink with the unwashed dishes, or strewn across the unmade beds? Were the answers in the hugs of my young children, or in their eye-rolls and impatient sighs? Were the answers in the disconnected relationships or the ones that continued to endure? Could they, in fact, be found on the scale or inside the label on my jeans?

The answer may surprise you.

Faith has always been a cornerstone in my life and therapy has not been too far behind. The laundry, the dishes, the beds – they all served a purpose but not MY purpose. The clues could be found in my relationships too, but not in a way you could imagine. While it is hard to admit, I believed for too long that the answers could be found on the scale or from that tiny little square inside my jeans.

It was none of these things.

I slowly began to realize that the thirst did not come from giving to others but was a result of not giving to myself. No matter how much was given to me, nothing could quench that thirst except when I gave to myself.

I am not talking about material things like clothes, or purses, or gifts for myself. I'm not even talking about pampering like pedicures, green drinks, or essential oils. It is not even found in date nights with my husband or nights out with friends. Although I enjoy those things, they nourish me in a much different way.

I am referring to practices and habits like listening to my body when it feels tired or hungry, praying when I am worried or fearful about the future, journaling to capture my thoughts or express the words I cannot verbalize, exercising or going for a walk when I feel stressed, giving myself permission to go to bed early or even stay up late.

One of the strongest ways to nourish myself is by exercising my ability to say no and being OK with using my voice—to express joy, silliness, anger, disappointment, relief, concern, fear, or boredom.

I find yet more empowerment through eating to nourish my body without self-criticism or judgment from others. I bolster my spirit by slowing down when the world yells, "FASTER!" I am finding the ways to stay true to myself in a society that yells, "FIT IN!" I am learning to tune in to the parts of myself where the gaps and the holes exist, parts of myself that I used to see as flaws, but now appreciate as unique things of beauty.

It is the practice of acknowledging and choosing the very things that make me, ME, just as you must acknowledge and choose the very things that make you, YOU.

Healing Begins Where the Light Shines Through

The Japanese practice that highlights and enhances flaws, thus adding value to a broken object, is called "kintsugi" (金継ぎ), literally golden ("kin") and repair ("tsugi"). The Kintsugi technique suggests many things, but the one thing I am sure of is that the essence of who you are is unique and precious, even in the midst of brokenness.

Healing your own brokenness takes time, patience and persistence, and can be accomplished in a myriad of ways. It is perhaps best summarized by Audrey Noble, "Self-care is the fight against the very thing that is hurting you by taking control of your own narrative; by looking inward to better negotiate the external."

The desert that I found myself in, the same desert you may be standing in right now, is not some arbitrary location you happened to stumble upon, but rather it is a direct accumulation of your habits, beliefs, and practices. And the water that you seek – the thirst that you long to quench – is not found on the scale.

Some people find their thirst is quenched through spiritual practices alone, while others find it is quenched through a combination of caring for themselves in mind, body and spirit. You decide what feels right for you.

Start by finding little ways that are meaningful to you, and align yourself with what matters most. It does not have to be an abrupt change, but rather a gentle shift. Pay attention to how your body feels, reflect on your thoughts, and make time to nourish your spirit.

Taking care of yourself does not mean, "Me first." It means, "Me, too." It does not mean that others are less important, rather it means that you are just as important. And if you are a parent, ask yourself, if you cannot show yourself love and acceptance, how can you teach it to your children?

Learning to love yourself is like learning to walk. It is not going to happen on the first try, and sometimes it is going to hurt. But just like a toddler beginning to take its first steps, the more you try, the more skilled you will become until one day, without a second thought, it will become a part of you.

Remind yourself that falling down is as much a part of the process as getting up, and when the inevitable happens, and you begin to leap for joy, you will scarcely remember life before you took your first tentative steps.

CHAPTER 5

Low Stress Investing

By Byron Harlan

Picture yourself in the most relaxed state possible. Maybe you hear birds. Maybe you're having the perfect massage, and there's no way you'll stay awake through the whole thing. That's exactly the state of mind I want you to achieve when it comes to investing. Sure, it's challenging, but attainable. It's a matter of achieving a mindset I call Zen Investing.

The securities markets do not have to be scary. With the right frame of mind, they can actually represent the opposite – a calm place, where investors can gain some measure of confidence. I'll share three stories with you to illustrate how approaching finances with your mind clear and your heart set on joyful interactions with loved ones can be a delightful way to lead your best life.

Money Fears and the Stock Market

You've probably heard the expression, "Timing is everything." It's an important proverb to keep in mind, especially when it comes to the sometimes bad and even disastrous decisions people make when they decide to get in and out of the securities markets. There may be no better evidence than what the markets return over time and what individual investors tend to earn, but, before this becomes a dull treatise about market timing, I'll share an anecdotal tale about the near panicked conversation I had recently with a prospective client.

The stress he was attempting to overcome was directly associated with the extreme volatility the stock market endured from the end of 2018, through the beginning of 2019. He could not stomach the ups-and-downs in his portfolio. I invited him for a visit, so we could discuss how to address his exposure to risk.

Ultimately, he decided that his strategy would be to run, wait until things had improved and then get re-invested. He was describing the very error so many people make: lock-in losses and limit gains which feeds into the panic-the-herd mentality that the financial media sometimes foster.

This stress can lead to bad decisions that have the potential to hurt your financial situation, which can increase stress even further and lock individuals into actions that were driven by anxiety.

Participation in the securities markets does not need to be a stressful endeavor. If you let them, they can be the source of a gratifying experience, enabling you to potentially out-pace inflation, retire comfortably, or establish a legacy for your heirs, if you wish.

I had the opportunity to appear on a radio program in early 2019, and I initiated the conversation with this question: Is it good, bad, or both when the stock market goes down?

The answer is both. Yet when commentators describe down markets, you'll sometimes hear this: "A bad day on Wall Street." One broadcaster called the massive Winter 2018 correction, "The worst week on Wall Street since 2008."

Think about the stress those words caused viewers who live on money they've invested in securities. It evokes memories of the major crash that happened roughly a decade earlier and paints the decline in a purely negative light.

It was quite the opposite for younger people, and I told my clients who were early in their accumulation years that the decline could be good news for them. It meant that they were essentially buying into the stock market at a discount. They listened, stuck with the strategy, and understood that when the correction ended, all those shares they bought during the contraction could reward them.

The same is not true for folks who are at or near retirement. A sharp decline can adversely impact their income, how long their portfolio will last, or both – which can be a readily available source of stress. The answer is a financial plan that addresses risk, which can involve a multitude of strategies designed to enable investors to retire comfortably and remain comfortably retired.

If you invest your dollars and sit tight, you will likely participate in a variety of market cycles, and you could come out ahead. The Dimensional Fund Advisors, 2018 Matrix Book reports that the 1926-to-2017 Standard & Poor's 500[1] index average yearly return was 10.2-percent. Let's all breathe and relax.

That brings us back to that prospective client who planned to flee the market. In this case, fear led to anxiety, which caused stress, which prompted retreat – a potentially costly sequence of emotions.

Editor's Note: In my health coaching practice, stress and overwork are two of the most common reasons that people overeat. The financial fears they harbor translate into stress, which then puts them on a path to working more to overcome the fear, but keeps them trapped in the cycle of work and stress. Therefore, I suggest

---

[1]The Standard & Poor's 500 (S&P 500) is a stock market index containing the stocks of 500 American corporations with large market capitalization that are considered to be widely held. Indexes cannot be invested in directly, are unmanaged, and do not incur management fees, costs and expenses. The information presented here should only be relied upon when coordinated with individual professional advice.

that addressing your finances should be part of your weight loss plan.

Planning Reduces Stress

Now breathe, relax, and, if you would, allow me to share a bit about another conversation I had recently with a friend.

It was impossible to miss his sorrow infused in a discussion I had recently with him. We were both born in 1959 and turned 60 in 2019. He was resigned that one of his most cherished material goals would be impossible to achieve. The dream was to own a particular style of home.

The dream itself seemed equally as important as the lesson that flowed from the exchange, because a strategy to fulfill his objective could have enabled him to acquire what he wanted. It was a stark reminder between the difference between planning and not doing so.

If it's apparent that a plan would have helped my friend to attain what he wanted, why did he not do so? That question sits somewhere on the mind of every good person who chooses to become a financial planner. What does it take for people to take that often pivotal step? What might be holding them back from developing a strategy to attain their dreams, then retire comfortably and stay comfortably retired?

Is it the desire to consume? Maybe, because, after all, how many people live paycheck-to-paycheck because of their desire to have what they want right now? My generation became infused with the values of the '80s. It was the norm to spend, acquire, and accumulate debt. It seemed easy to ignore the cost of what you wanted in exchange for the rush that came with getting something new.

How many folks eat out, spend more than they should and throw-down a heavily worn credit card to pay for it?

Here's something to consider: Say you spend five-dollars a day for a fancy coffee drink and ten-dollars a day for lunch. That comes to about 450-dollars a month. If instead you invested in a moderate to aggressive portfolio, the total, after 20-years, could be around $230,000. Maybe it would be better to brew coffee at home and pack lunch most days.

Editor's Note: You may have goals and values that align with making your lunch at home and saving money to invest. When you are under continual stress, as I see in my health coaching practice that so many of us are, that stress sabotages your ability to make long-term decisions.

When stress hormones kick in, they drive you to get the take out or the sweet coffee drink, even if your mind is saying not to. Stress is often a cause for short sighted decisions; stress is also a leading cause of weight gain. Once again, it is essential to look at ways to manage your stress so that you can make the decisions that serve you long term, for your finances as well as your health.

Another deep breath here might help.

Yes, it takes money to hire a Financial Planner[2], but how much? What's it worth to find out when you can stop working and not run out of money? My partner and I have structured our practice so

---

[2] It is common for financial planners to carry a designation. Many people are familiar with the letters, CFP ®, which stand for CERTIFIED FINANCIAL PLANNER™ There are others too. Mine is the RICP ®, Retirement Income Certified Professional ® and I'm about halfway through the CFP ® curriculum. My wife and business partner holds the ChFC ®, which stands for Chartered Financial Consultant ®. She recently completed work on her BFA™ designation, short for Behavioral Financial Advice. These designations, and others, indicate that the person who earned them has acquired a unique set of skills.

that the assets we manage cover the cost to develop a financial plan for clients.

We did it this way because we believe it's extremely valuable for folks to have a game-plan together. Whether or not you work with us, we believe it's useful to work with someone to design a plan to help you get what you want, which sometimes includes the money for a particular style of home that you've always desired.

My 60-year-old friend is lucky; he's in a profession that could enable him to work another 15-years or more. It's possible that he can achieve his dream, with the proper planning. The only question is will he develop a plan or not? My hope is that he will. I want things to go well for my friend so that he can accomplish his dreams. Wish me luck in convincing him it's possible, when I speak with him again.

The Bigger Picture

I often say that money and the pursuit of it cannot and should not be a top priority. You're not defined by your net worth; you're defined by the love you give. That may sound strange coming from a Financial Planner, but the experiences I had with my mother during the winter of 2018 and 2019 provided the truth for what I believe.

Instead of the typically overflowing joy in my home during the holidays, there was a heaviness because of my mother's failing health. My mother had received a diagnosis from a neurologist, confirming she had both Alzheimer's and Parkinson's. Our family is doing everything possible to slow the onset of these two debilitating diseases, but the progression is inevitable. It is tragic and horrible.

One winter day we went out to lunch. I hoped that she could provide – just one more time – the precious advice that she'd given me through the years. When times were tough, she used to say, "This too shall pass." She would also say, "Talk to God." She would reassure me that things would be OK, in a way that only a mother can.

This time, it was different. When I talked about my challenges, the difficulties of running my own practice and the weight of the responsibilities I felt, I saw a lost look in her eyes. There were no warm, loving words, just a distant, somewhat confused appearance about her, as her eyes drifted from me to the other patrons in the restaurant and around the room. It was heartbreaking.

Thankfully, our family had the means to move her to a home where she could receive exceptional care. When the time came, though, one of the owners said it would be best to not see her for the first two weeks of her stay, so she could become acclimated. That first visit was emotional, intense, and wonderful.

I could not hold back the tears, when I paid my mother her first visit in her new memory care home. I cried on her shoulder, told her, "I love you," and she responded with the same beautiful words. We held hands and talked a bit before she said to me, "Go home and get some rest." It was a moment when things felt as they always had, and I cherished it.

My plea to you is this: Value your loved ones, your health, and your dreams; they are more important than material aspirations. Too much of what I see is connected with the material goals of consumption: what to buy, how much money to have and hold.

We jockey for parking spaces to rush into stores, so we can spend and acquire possessions that, ultimately, become meaningless one day. We try to outsmart the securities markets or seek "hot" stocks to grow a pile of money for the sake of a larger pile of money. We envy what others have and too often cause personal financial strain to obtain what someone else possesses.

The energy devoted to these endeavors is misplaced. I believe the core of what matters includes family, experiences, dreams, joy, and health. So, my message to you is not about portfolio performance, nor mutual fund recommendations. We can carve out plenty of time for that.

My message is simply this: Love the precious people in your life as much as you can, while you can, and while they're around to receive it.

It is important to note that all investing involves risk, including the potential loss of principal. Past performance cannot guarantee future results. Current performance may be lower or higher. No investment strategy can guarantee a profit or protect against loss. Please note that individual situations can vary.

The opinions expressed here are those of the author; therefore, the information presented in this chapter should not be construed as investment advice. Byron Harlan is a Financial Planner and offers Securities through Royal Alliance Associates, Inc. (RAA), member FINRA/SIPC, and Investment Advisory services through NWF Advisory Services, who is not affiliated with RAA. 1240 India St., #1402, San Diego, CA, 92101. 619-400-4994. CA Insurance License #0G31264. bharlan@royalaa.com

Part 2: Putting It Together

Replacing the Old Beliefs with Healthy Habits

CHAPTER 6

Emotional Well-Being and Boundaries

By Melissa Rosenstock

People tend to focus more on their physical health — eating nutritious foods, drinking plenty of water, exercising, and getting enough sleep — to achieve optimal health, and while it is important to pay attention to it, lasting success requires a more holistic approach.

Stimulating your mind and nourishing yourself on a soulful or spiritual level are also critical components to your overall well-being, yet too often they are not factored into the well-being equation.

You can follow a diet and exercise regime and see results, but if your neglect your emotional well-being, your success will be temporary. All the kale and exercise will not make up for nourishing your emotional well-being.

I like to cluster the pillars of well-being into five core categories: Physical Health, Emotional Health, Relationships (family, spouse/partner, friends, colleagues), Vocation (career or job as well as other ways you develop and share your skills), and Finances. Looking at these holistically is fundamental. It is the body, mind, and soul integration which comprise your overall well-being, and how they work together determines how you feel.

Physical & Emotional Well-being

It is one thing to know the significance of the pillars and essentials that comprise your well-being yet it is another to understand the potential impact each one has and adjust accordingly. At the core is your emotional well-being and physical well-being. Although separate entities, they are intertwined.

Your emotional health affects your physical health and vice versa. When you are feeling depressed, angry or irritable, or simply in a funk, then "symptoms" begin to show up in your physical body, whether it be digestive issues, tiredness, or headaches, to name only a few. Synergy between your emotional health and your physical health impacts your well-being as a whole.

How do you nourish your emotional well-being? By feeding your soul — going deeper into yourself to find what brings you joy, peace, contentment, and overall fulfillment. Soul nourishment is personalized. When it comes to your well-being, there will never be a one-size-fits-all plan.

What comes before anything is defining what soul nourishment is for you. Maybe it is lacing up your running shoes and heading out the door for an early morning jog; or taking your journal to sit with your thoughts, while sitting on the beach and listening to the waves crash against the sand; or laughing with friends and catching up with them over dinner; or maybe it is curling up on the couch to devour a new book, with a steaming cup of hot tea to warm you.

Soul nourishment has no limits. You get to decide what it is, and you may notice that it dips between both worlds — the emotional and physical, further proving how they are woven together, and how they actually feed one another.

When you are not starving the emotional side of your well-being, but are actually feeding it exactly what it needs to thrive, then it manifests on the physical side. The by-product of feeding your emotional well-being may translate to weight loss.

Your emotional well-being holds the key to your desires — be it weight loss or simply feeling good in body, mind, and soul. It is critical to heed to your emotional needs as much, if not more than, your physical needs. Your body needs water and food to survive, as your emotions need nutrition for the soul.

If you feed your body with poor food and drink and do not exercise, then your physical body will suffer greatly, which will bleed into your emotional well-being too. Quality nutrients and moving your body are a great boost to your physical and emotional well-being, but the next step is to feed and exercise your inner well-being.

Many people are quick to diminish or ignore their emotions. What you are not willing to address or work through can be detrimental to your health. It may be easier to focus on food and exercise, because those are controllable and the outcome may be clearer, however, emotional turmoil is less predictable.

It can be difficult to confront emotions that have been at bay for months, or perhaps even years, but with clarity come benefits.

There are no shortcuts. The only way around it is directly through it. The greater the challenge, the bigger the gift. The gift lies within you. That gift is freedom from the inner and emotional turmoil that is standing in the way of where you want to be right now.

The distance between where you are and where you want to be may not be as far as you think. Your thoughts either widen or close the gap. The most powerful tool is your mind which is either telling you, "Yes, you can," or "No, you can't."

In reality, neither is true until you give your thoughts power to believe one over the other. Henry Ford succinctly stated, "Whether you think you can or think you can't, you're right."

Your thoughts persuade you to follow a certain path. Your capabilities are limited by your thoughts, unless you choose to think you are limitless. Thoughts, while extremely powerful, must be coupled with action and belief to achieve your goals.

Can your thoughts lead to weight loss? Partially, because your thoughts need to precede action. Thoughts alone will not make you thin, but when you believe and envision yourself losing weight, feeling healthy, and wearing clothes that make you feel good, then you begin to take the actions that perpetuate weight loss.

Spend time envisioning what you want and believing it can happen, to the point that you feel it. Embody the feelings you desire, then the outcome becomes realized by your belief in the vision.

When you embody what you want before you have it, then you take the actions to match that which you desire. You begin to make the choices that are in direct alignment with the person you are envisioning yourself to already be.

Boundaries

When presented with food choices, exercise options, and other lifestyle alternatives, it comes down to one thing. Most people think it is determined by willpower and that is a myth. It has nothing to do with your will and everything to do with boundaries. How does this look in reality?

Setting boundaries are critical to your success — whether it be with weight loss, relationships, career, or time management, every area of your life is impacted by the boundaries you set in place.

Beyond creating boundaries, adhering to the boundaries you set will be a crucial aspect that will carry you to success.

Boundaries are not meant to be restrictive because your body and mind will immediately resist. Boundaries pull you in the direction you want to go, where restriction pushes you where you don't want to be, creating friction. That friction of resistance keeps you stuck, furthering the distance between where you are and where you want to be.

When you set boundaries without being too restrictive, then you provide a framework that is not only doable, but sustainable. With anything you implement in your life, especially when creating new habits, sustainability is key.

If it is not something you see yourself doing long term, then your success will be temporary. This is why undue restricting is not a sustainable practice.

Why are boundaries so important? They act as a guiding force when there are numerous options and opportunities. Boundaries are linked to what you are aiming to achieve.

You are the driver and the boundaries become the GPS guiding you to your destination, your goals. If you don't know where you're headed, then you can't set your GPS.

How can you set practical boundaries without restrictions that you can adhere to and implement in your daily life? As mentioned earlier, the first step is to know the goal — whether it is weight loss, healthier living, or simply prioritizing your needs. Then you will have a guide to determine if a decision is aligned with your desired outcome.

If weight loss is your goal, then you set boundaries around what you will and will not keep in the house, providing a framework for success to be actualized. It is not about saying, "I will never eat cake again."

Not only is that too restrictive, but it is not realistic or sustainable over time. It is about creating goals that serve your well-being without depriving yourself.

For example, when you go to a restaurant, and are presented with a multitude of options, the boundaries you've set act as the guide for what choice best supports your goal, keeping it top of mind.

Support

When you are embarking on a personal development journey, it is important to have support. Share with your loved ones your goals and why it is important for you to make healthy changes. Also share with those around you, such as colleagues and co-workers. Including others enables them to support you as desired. Often, people want to help, but they are not always sure how to do so.

However, if co-workers and family are not supportive, you need not force it or take it personally. People may be down on things they are not willing to do for themselves.

If you don't find the support you need from the people you are closest with, then seek support elsewhere — be it with friends, at the gym, or investing in a coach. A coach can provide the framework you need and hold you accountable to help you reach your goals.

By sharing with your loved ones your undertaking to improve your well-being, then they can offer support in helping you to protect and enforce the boundaries you've set.

If your best friend, mom, and/or spouse see you respecting the boundaries you've put in place for yourself, then they're not going to convince you to eat the French fries, skip your workout, and drown your worries in a bottle of champagne.

On the contrary, they will be the ones to encourage and support your healthy endeavors, helping you to strengthen your healthy boundaries. Perhaps you'll even influence others to take care of themselves when they see the positive change in you.

Why do you want what you want? This is an important question to answer. The "why" is what fuels the process, aligns you to your boundaries, and what drives you towards your goal. Look beyond a number on the scale or a certain dress size, and instead focus upon how you want to feel. What does the number mean to you? What would shift if you sought a feeling instead of a number?

For example, how might you feel when you slip into your favorite pair of jeans and catch a positive glimpse of yourself in the mirror, or how might you feel when you walk up a flight of stairs without stopping to catch your breath. Feelings are far more powerful and important than numbers.

Becoming fixated on a number can render you powerless in your pursuit to achieve it. On the contrary, when you put your focus on a desired feeling, then the power is within your control.

How can you create an environment that breeds your ability to thrive across all pillars of well-being?

- Know your why, your reason for wanting what you desire. Once you are committed to it, then it becomes the driving force propelling you forward.
- Write down your intentions including your why, your vision, your goals, and your desired feelings. Be super specific!
- Create and adhere to boundaries that are aligned with your intentions.

- Ask for support and build a network that will help you along the way.
- Nourish and feed your soul. Find what lights you up, brings you joy, and fuels you.

Word Choice Matters

Words also matter, whether directed towards others or yourself. Kindness is key. When you become aware of your thoughts and how they affect your actions, then you can make different choices.

If you are constantly spewing negative thoughts towards yourself and being ultra-critical, then your progress will be thwarted. Negative thoughts and being unkind to yourself breeds a stagnant environment where you cannot grow and thrive.

"I've been bad today." Have you ever uttered those words where diet is concerned? Food choices do not make you a bad or good person. By nature, you are an inherently good person, and deciding to have dessert when you told yourself you wouldn't does not make you a bad person.

You can rephrase it to "I did not make the best choice for myself today." Your words can have a lasting effect, and this simple shift in word choice will have a direct and positive impact on your well-being and your progress. Kind words foster the confidence to adhere to the boundaries you've set for yourself.

While all concepts in this chapter are important components to your success, none is more so than this one decision: deciding to prioritize yourself for the sake of your well-being. Nothing will change if you do not choose to put yourself on your own radar.

If you spend all of your time and energy putting others' needs before your own, then you have nothing left to give to yourself. Putting your needs on the back burner will cost you your health and well-being. Before you do anything, decide that your well-being is a top priority.

When you prioritize yourself, and follow it with thoughts and actions that support your decision, then you are sending a signal that creates a mind-body-soul connection. Once that connection has been put into play, then you have put yourself on the path to well-being.

By making your health a priority, then making better choices where food, exercise, and lifestyle are concerned, the process becomes infinitely easier. What you affirm or deny is at the forefront of your awareness because you have chosen to prioritize yourself.

Your emotional well-being and your mindset are the most critical components to your achievement! An attitude of kindness will move you closer to your goal faster than any negative thought will, whereas criticism and negative self-talk moves you further away from where you want to be.

How can you offer yourself kindness with your words, your thoughts, and your actions? One kind word can change the trajectory of your day and maybe even your life, so can you give that to yourself?

There is no one diet or exercise program that works for everyone. It is about finding what you like to do, and what is the most sustainable over the long term. At the end of the day, it has to feel pleasurable. Sometimes it may feel uncomfortable and challenging, and that is okay. Growth does not happen from doing the same things you've always done.

So, there is a certain level of moving out of your comfort zone that needs to take place, and challenging yourself, which may not always feel comfortable. Discomfort does not mean feeling bad.

Remind yourself that feeling uncomfortable is temporary and focus on your goal to move through it, coming out the other side to feeling good.

Diet and exercise may not be one-size-fits-all, but mindset is universal. A mindset of self-supporting, positive thoughts and most importantly, beliefs, works. You have to believe your goals are possible. When you believe in yourself and embody the beliefs, then you are establishing a mindset of possibility and faith.

You are creating the pathway to your success through the power of your thoughts, beliefs and actions. It all starts with one thought, one belief, and one action. What is one step you can take today to move you closer to your goal? Believe!

CHAPTER 7

Weight Loss Basics

By Alegra Loewenstein

It is essential to cover a few basics that are often overlooked by those wishing to lose weight.

As you have seen in other chapters of this book, the most important mindset shift is honoring yourself. One of the most essential ways to honor your body and set protective boundaries starts with the absolute basics of healthcare.

Stress

The human body is incredibly robust and adaptable. Unfortunately, one of the few things that our bodies cannot withstand is chronic stress. Evolutionarily stress is designed to be short-term; think running from a saber toothed cat or hunting some wild deer. But in the 21st century stress is everywhere.

Even what you do for fun, spending time on your computer and phone, is actually a form of stress. Not all screens are bad, but they can induce stress hormones when you spend a prolonged time on your devices (and you can give yourself a "hit" of these stress hormones by glancing briefly at your phone).

So, we think we will lie down on the sofa and relax, but we end up looking at our phone. We feel re-energized, but that's actually because of stress hormones. We are essentially self-medicating with stress hormones around the clock, and then we wonder why we can't sleep. I say we, because I still struggle! For me, I end up with neck pain and headaches, both caused by insufficient or disrupted sleep.

My neck is my "canary in the mine." What is yours? Perhaps it is your weight. In this way, your body is telling you it can't handle the situation anymore. Managing stress is something everyone in the 21st century has to come to terms with. Your body informs you how stress is affecting you, and it's time to listen.

Managing your stress and setting up healthy boundaries and expectations is a theme throughout this book. That's because it is essential to successful weight loss. If you don't manage your stress, then you will not lose weight. It may sound harsh, but stress actually causes our bodies to retain weight.

It is responsible, in particular, for weight gain around the abdominal area. This is one of the most difficult regions to lose your weight. That is because, in most cases of stubborn weight around your core, you have not managed your stress. No amount of exercise can resolve this predicament.

Exercise is an absolutely wonderful way to reduce stress. But if you don't have basic boundaries in place, then adding exercise on top of your already stressed life actually causes additional stress. Exercise creates healthy hormones, but at the same time requires a time commitment in an already busy schedule. Something has to give!

Identifying the causes of your stress is essential. Maybe the answer is obvious to you or there might be additional causes of stress that you're unaware of, which require more contemplation.

Failure to let go of stress can also complicate matters. For example, maintaining toxic relationships can adversely affect stress level. Some feel an undue sense of obligation, whether with friends or family. If people are unnecessarily causing you stress, then it is time to be brutally honest with yourself about its cost.

If the time has come to free yourself from a relationship, honor your feelings of grief, loss, sadness, or failure. Create space to process the change through therapy, journaling, or ritual. Give yourself the gift of a life free from people who drag you down and drain your energy.

A second common form of stress is that from work, which is the most common type that my clients encounter. Sometimes it is harder to deal with because while it may cause stress, you may also enjoy your work or are obliged to earn money. You may not be able to change your situation quickly.

However, it is essential to move through the steps that will alleviate the stress. The first step is to acknowledge that the stress is a problem. The second step is to expand your awareness about how it is affecting you, looking at what triggers your stress.

The third step is implement boundaries that begin to shield you from the stress. The fourth step is to integrate tiny changes (turning off notifications or leaving on time, for example). The fifth (and recurring) step is to reassess and add more small changes.

Sleep

Ahhhh. Sleep. This is the healthcare basic that everybody wants to ignore. As a society, we do not value sleep! The omnipresent pressures of our modern world are constantly eating into a good night of rest. But, just like stress, if you are short on sleep consistently, no other health care or weight loss effort will matter.

Sleep deprivation will cause your body to retain weight. Lack of sleep, even chronically getting just half an hour or an hour less than you need, will cause hormonal disruptions that make it nearly impossible to reach your ideal natural weight. So to lose weight, you have to get ample quality sleep.

It will take time and dedication. It will take shifting the small habits that are eroding away at your sleep. It may mean leaving that last email unsent. It may mean leaving that laundry soaking in the washer to dry in the morning. It means releasing a million little things that you used to do before going to bed.

Also, there is an opportunity to outsource. Bringing in more support can be liberating. This can cover a wide range of items, such as:

- household help
- cleaning
- yard work
- In home chef
- virtual assistant to reply to routine emails
- getting more things delivered
- more childcare/babysitting
- professional organizer
- personal trainer
- planned workout program

Take time to assess your trusted helpers. It took a few tries to find someone that I completely trust with house cleaning, but she was worth the wait! I happily pay her more , because she is a welcome presence in my home who brings joy and peace.

I write her thank you notes a few times a year and give her an end of year bonus from the bottom of my heart. Look for a relationship that will spark that kind of joy.

Finances can be a constraint. Ask yourself how much you might spend in a year on protein powders, books, programs, and other weight loss items you may be tempted to try. You will be buying less of the "magic bullet" items (that of course won't really solve the problem).

That money can now be redirected for outsourcing chores that cause you stress and cut into your sleep time, knowing you are getting to the root of the problem.

Ask yourself what your health is worth long term, and invest to bring your life into balance. Project into the future to speculate what neglecting your health might cost you if your health declines and you develop chronic problems.

This is an opportunity to assess your goals and values and possibly reassess how you align your financial values with your life values.

This problem has many creative solutions. Clients have paid their teenage children to do the majority of the household chores redirecting the money while increasing support from their family at the same time.

Other clients who know industrious teens in their neighborhood, hire them for a variety of household tasks, from basic computer work to housecleaning. Others rebalance housework with a partner which costs nothing and relieves stress (and reduces resentment). Brainstorm new ideas for your home!!

When you decide health is your priority, it's natural to witness a ripple effect through various aspects of your life to support this. Getting more sleep support health and weight loss. Making changes in how you spend your time and money support getting more sleep (and reduce stress). There are many pathways you can take to create this change in your life. Have fun while you find the ones that work best for you.

Alcohol

Alcohol consumption can also affect health. Although I don't advocate abstinence, consistent drinking causes weight gain and other problems. You probably know that, too. It's OK to enjoy a drink with friends or family on the weekends. I give you permission to enjoy indulgences, and I advise you enjoy them in moderation.

So, how do we avoid the overindulging trap? It's only Wednesday, and that glass of wine sounds sounds enticing. Imagining a glass of wine in your hand conjures a temptation of changing gears with ease, unwinding at the end of your busy day, and treating yourself to something special and enjoyable.

If one glass often turns into two or three, and just tonight turns into most of the week, you're suddenly consuming a lot of calories and refined sugars. Of course, excessive alcohol consumption can also cause weight gain and hormonal imbalances complicating weight loss. Using alcohol as a coping mechanism also means you'll continue the patterns that make you want to drink in the first place.

Two secrets to regulating alcohol consumption are to assess your stress level and personal values in order to avoid self-sabotage. It's simple, but it's not always easy. This will require you to find other ways to relax. Even if healthier habits are inconvenient, they will serve you long-term. New rituals will enhance your daily life.

Water

We all know we need to stay hydrated but may not be aware of its effect on weight loss. It is common to think you are hungry when you are actually thirsty!

Additionally, because stress is often correlated with weight gain, it's also common to consume large amounts of caffeine in tea or coffee or soda, but caffeine can also be a diuretic so it is not as beneficial as water.

There are conflicting arguments about how much water a person needs. While some suggest eight 8-ounce glasses per day (64 ounces per day total), others argue that you need half your weight in ounces (example: If you weigh 180 pounds, you should drink 90 ounces of water per day).

At the other end of the spectrum is to drink when you feel thirsty; since a majority of people in modern society do not pay attention to their bodies' signals, this results in as little as 8-32 ounces of water per day for most people, which is insufficient.

Personally, I strive for the middle ground of six to eight 8-ounce glasses in a day. If I drink less than six glasses in a day, I can tell. (However, I don't beat myself up if I drink less.)

One simple trick to stay hydrated is to figure out how many of your water bottles you need to drink in a day to get ample water. Alternatively, when I'm home, I prefer to use a beautiful glass pitcher.

Happy Chemicals

Another theme in this book is the effect of hormones or, more accurately, a combination of hormones and neurotransmitters. Don't worry, you don't need to know the difference to know how to improve your situation.

Basically, hormones (such as adrenaline, oxytocin, melatonin, insulin) and neurotransmitters (such as dopamine, serotonin) and also endorphins are the "happy chemicals" that make us feel good. Balancing these happy chemicals creates sustained energy and well-being and lifts moods.

However, when these chemicals become imbalanced, it can cause problems. A sole chemical can become imbalanced, or it can cause a chain reaction. It's a sophisticated and complex interplay that is easily disrupted by stress, poor nutrition, or a sedentary lifestyle.

The result is that eating makes us feel happy temporarily because it releases endorphins, but when it's the primary source of our happy chemicals, it becomes unsustainable.

Another common scenario is stress that produces happy chemicals, too, but that actually depletes us over time, and usually stimulates us to seek food again, which traps us in old habits that prohibit us from attaining our goals!

Without realizing it, we can become addicted to these habits, continually seeking the release of happy chemicals, despite the fact that we feel bad after the initial benefit.

Sometimes we can identify the source of the troublesome habit, such as too much alcohol or not enough sleep, but more often it's a combination of factors. However, steps to bring one happy chemical into balance bring them all into balance!

For example, even if lack of sleep isn't a problem, getting abundant sleep will still help restore your body, so that it can efficiently do the job of balancing all the happy chemicals, naturally.

Happy chemicals, habits, mood, self care, and self worth are all intricately intertwined. To establish balance, you must first see yourself as worthy, then take care of yourself, which will lift your mood, which will lead to healthier habits, which brings your happy chemicals into balance. Tiny steps lead to your well-being.

These are the absolute health care basics for success when it comes to weight loss. With minimal effort, your body can reach its ideal natural weight.

If staying on track feels overwhelming or impossible, be honest with yourself and seek support. Don't waste your money on a magic bullet; there is no such thing. It's not about what's fastest, it's about gradual change that creates a paradigm shift.

Support comes in various forms such as a health coach or even family and friends to provide accountability, encouragement, praise, and personalized fresh ideas. Who will make healthy choices with you?

Can you change that coffee date with your friend to meet for a walk instead? Can your brother or sister bring a green salad to the next family event? Perhaps a great book will bring you the focus you need. A guided journal can be a perfect way to start. (You can also review my list for ideas to outsource.)

If you have indulged in extreme deprivation diets or binge diets or crash diets, your metabolism may be altered and may take extra work to restore it.

The upcoming food chapter suggests basic approaches to nutrition that, in conjunction with this basic health foundation, will balance your metabolism as well. Ask your medical provider for further guidance.

The secret to lasting weight loss really does exist in your mindset. You did not get stuck where you are in 21 days. You didn't get here in 30 days. It wasn't even 12 weeks of imbalance. It took months and even years. Restoring your body's natural weight will not happen in days or weeks. If you lose weight quickly, you're going to gain it back.

Instead, you need to focus on the bigger picture. It may take six months or a year or longer to make sure the weight you lose stays off. Small steps of self-care that honor your values can result in feeling better immediately.

Drinking eight cups of water as a radical act of loving yourself can feel awesome and will energize you to do it again! Small steps can make big magic! You're not just losing weight. You are crafting a life that sparkles!

CHAPTER 8

Yoga Awareness for a Balanced Life

By David Sonsara

Changing a mindset is no easy project. Fulfilling daily requirements for food, shelter, and comfort may easily result in automatic behaviors. Interactions with others during meals, on the job, or during activities often become habitual.

Habits aren't always negative; they can help our mind function more efficiently. Pondering every decision would be too time consuming! However, unhealthy habits can result in pain or limited motion, a more sedentary life, and ultimately extra weight.

Although changing our mindset may not be easy, the solution may be as simple as watching yourself breathe.

Watch Yourself Breathe, Change Your Habits

Watching your breath can create awareness of how your body and mind interact. When you breathe and pay attention to interactions between your body and mind, there is an awakening of opportunities to grow and change your set mind. Over time, monitoring our breathing can expand our self-awareness across many aspects of our lives.

As Dennis Waitley said, "The truth is, you don't break a bad habit, you replace it with a good one." Mindful breathing can be a useful way to start a good habit (and replace a bad habit).

We all have challenges in our lives, which can be bubbling at the surface or rumbling deeper inside, even after numerous attempts to correct the problems. Some problems appear to be more urgent.

However, by tuning into your body through deep breathing, you'll begin to expand awareness of how urgent the problem truly is, going beyond your initial bodily reaction, which may feel stronger than warranted.

Overreaction and obsession can put our perspective off balance. My daily practice of mindful breathing calms me during stressful doctor and dentist appointments, helping me realize they are part of normal modern life, despite the anxiety I may sometimes feel.

When overreacting to a problem, we may wonder if resolution is even possible! I suggest looking for a way to evolve the situation, as opposed to resolve the problem.

This simple shift in language can open up possibilities, compared the single-minded focus of resolving or "fixing a problem, which can feel overwhelming. If you can "evolve," you may find a broader approach and more balanced life.

Balancing life includes recognition that life is not only about resolving hardships but also acknowledging the best in life. To this end, monitoring my breath while performing piano for an audience has expanded my sense of joy and peace. Living to the fullest acknowledges both concerns and accomplishments, sorrow and joy within a balanced life.

Observe Your Body

The mind directs the body, both consciously and unconsciously, and impacts every aspect of life. Our beliefs direct our intentions. Transforming unconscious to conscious breathing promotes the mind-body connection.

With eyes s*lightly* closed, observe the quality of your breath as you breathe deeply while relaxing for a few moments. This simple action tunes you in to what in yoga is called your "mind's eye" or the "third eye" – a feeling of awareness that expands beyond plain sight and improves awareness for a more balanced life.

While continuing to observe deeper breathing from your stomach, reflect upon your concerns for another few minutes. Notice what you feel and where, consciously revealing the body's physical response when your mind focuses on your concerns. If you observe tension somewhere, allow your third eye to watch the deep breath relax that part of your body.

This conscious connection between your body's physical response and the subjects that cross your mind becomes useful in "evolving" through the concerns. Full deep breaths activate the soothing parasympathetic nervous system. With a calm mind, fresh perspectives emerge. Short-term and long-term intentions begin to find balance within life's bigger picture.

The seemingly urgent obstacles may fade to the background, so you can see the bigger picture more clearly. Long held concerns may loosen their grip. When the mind becomes conscious of physical responses to our worries and stress, we can employ intentional change. As Deepak Chopra has simply stated, "What I am aware of, I can change."

Whatever your physical response may be – a knot in the stomach, tightness in the chest, hunched shoulders, grinding teeth – mindful breathing can release tension. Monitoring our breathing is the first step of mapping the mind-body connection.

This map is a tool to understand how the mind and body interact as one: the mind-body. The map directs us how to increase our awareness of how a balanced mind-body feels.

The mind-body maps identify the zones that are out of balance. Pain in our bodies, whether it's back pain, neck pain, knee pain or elsewhere, is usually caused or magnified by imbalance. Having awareness of the mind-body map can identify the source of the imbalance that is causing pain.

Physically, the mind-body map has slowly improved my awareness of balancing my hips and heart. Once you are aware of the imbalance, you can make changes and live more freely with less pain.

Creating awareness of your body through this mind-body map will improve your range of motion through the release of physical tension with mindful breathing. Body movement will be discussed further in the next section. First, let's create some structure for our map of the mind-body connection.

Three Zones in Your Mind and Body

To understand mapping the mind to the body, we will examine three zones in the body:

- Hips
- Heart
- Head

This simple concept can give you an idea of how your body is responding to what you are thinking and experiencing. As you practice deep, slow breaths, check in with what you are feeling in each of the three zones: First the hips and legs, then the heart and trunk, then the head and neck. Which area is tight? Where you do you feel tension? Is there pain in any of the areas?

These zones apply to both our physical body as well as our mental/emotional existence. In modern day society, we live in our heads, and this manifests itself in our head forward posture, hunched shoulders, and rounded upper back.

Living in our heads promotes disconnect from our bodies, and it also keeps us living with the "fight or flight" sympathetic nervous system continuously activated. Physical energy is wastefully spent holding on to this tension!

Breathing releases the tension and frees up locked energy for other uses. A balanced body allows the hips, heart, and head zones to move more easily through full range of motion in three ways: from front to back, side to side, and twisting rotation.

When all three directions are combined, your body can move through full range of motion. Think of moving in circles!

Additionally, from the hips, the legs move in all three directions; from the heart, the arms move in all three directions; and holding up the head, the spine moves in all three directions. We need to balance heart and hips in order to balance our tendency to be in our head. Balancing our body makes us aware of our day-to-day habits.

I consciously make adjustments to balance my hips before exercising or walking or strengthening weaker muscles. Despite having arthritis in my hip, my awareness and conscious effort to balance these three zones has, over time, allowed me to regain mobility and strength.

When we explore new body movements, we must find a balance between push and pull. At the edge of our comfort, hold it, melting that edge, softening that tightness, before we retreat into the safety of what was already comfortable.

You can become aware of this simple edge the next time you stretch any muscle: When you reach the edge of the stretch, hold it for forty seconds without pushing, then relax. See if you don't go a bit further into the stretch, as you begin to melt those edges.

As always, this applies to both our physical body as well as our spirit. As we create new habits, new awareness through our breath, it can feel uncomfortable, even scary. We have to stay in that awareness, with our eyes closed, allowing ourselves to breathe, even as our old habits tell us to open our eyes and react to our passing emotions.

How to Think About Chakras

Next, we will learn how these three zones connect to the seven energy centers within the body known as chakras. Chakras are defined by Merriam-Webster as "any of several points of physical or spiritual energy in the human body according to yoga philosophy."

Using chakras to think about how energy moves through your body and connects with your emotions, mind, and spirit will create opportunities for awareness that may lead to a more peaceful and joyful life.

Far from being woo-woo or "out there," this simple practice of awareness of your body actually grounds you in living the values that are most important to you. It also helps locked energy along the spine to be freed for other intentions How great is that?

Whether you prefer to talk about the three zones of the body or have an extensive knowledge of the chakras, the zones and names are tools to bring awareness to what is happening in your body. Remember that what is most important is that you use your awareness – whether from breathing or movement – to breathe into the tight places. We name the elements only to make connections through our mind-body map and direct the body in new ways.

Next, I'll introduce the chakras from bottom to top – from earth to sky:

Hips: 1st STABILITY – the pelvic floor

2nd CREATIVITY – between the navel and the pubic bone

Heart: 3rd POWER – at the base of the sternum/breastbone

4th HEART – at the top of the sternum/breastbone

Head: 5th TRUTH – at the throat

6th INTUITION – the mind's eye (between eyebrows)

7th AWARENESS – the crown of the head

Chakras are tools to further the mapping of the mind-body connection, which improves the quality of awareness and promotes feeling balanced in both the mind and the body.

Take some time now to recall what you felt as your mind's eye (the intuitive 6th chakra) was observing your concerns and breath earlier. Return to observing several deep breaths now if needed.

Make note of where you feel tension or what you are thinking about; look at the simple chakra list, and identify either the area of the body or the key word (in capital letters) that you associate with your observations.

There is no wrong answer, this is simply helping you expand your awareness. After identifying your feeling on the chakra map, set your intention for the changes you desire. You may wish to write down what you felt, in which zone or chakra, and how you may use this information to make a small positive change in your life.

We first become aware of imbalances, then we watch the evolution, intentionally taking steps to improve balanced awareness. Practicing watching yourself breath will provide information from your body that your mind can use to move toward new results.

Using the Map in Your Everyday

Watching life through the eyes of our body as well as our mind promotes a fresh perspective on life. Your mind-body map is simply a more detailed version of your mind-body connection. The map, whether through the three zones or the seven chakras, brings heightened awareness and knowledge, and empowers you to release stress and improve balance throughout the whole of life.

Use the calming power mindful breathing to change habits, and use the mind-body map to reach your long-term intentions. Our pure awareness expands without limits; there is always something new to observe or learn or change. What the mind's eye focuses on will continuously evolve.

As George Bernard Shaw said, "Progress is impossible without change, and those who cannot change their minds cannot change anything"

Changing our mind is always an option, even if challenging. Often, our mind is so busy talking we forget to listen to our body. Watching our breath helps us learn to listen to the body by refocusing the inner voice. By creating this mind-body connection, we can calm both, and we can change both. Our breath brings awareness, and awareness brings change.

CHAPTER 9

Movement as Play

By Maggie Paola

Changing your perspective about exercise can be like turning a massive ship in the ocean. A paradigm shift is required to understand that movement is much more than just exercise. It's more than working out. It's more than training. It's more than lifting weights.

Movement is *playing, running, twirling, jumping, dancing, wriggling, stretching and much more*: Movement is all the words children think of as playing. This is the necessary paradigm shift. Stop thinking of struggling at the gym, and start having fun like when you were a child (or as your own children do). All that is needed is a swing and slide, and life is enjoyable!

Watch a child at a playground. They're filled with delight to climb up a ladder, and slide down. Wheeeeee! Movement is a natural part of life. Moving our body can be fun. How do you like to move?

- Dancing (Turn on your favorite music, go to a good concert!)
- Tennis
- Volleyball
- Gymnastics
- Basketball
- Soccer
- Ballet

- Hiking
- Swimming
- Surfing

As "grown ups," we often limit what we do to what we know we're good at, and we rarely venture into trying new sports or activities. Why risk a bike ride, when we can be safe and warm in our car? Usually parents let their children experiment with different sports and hobbies. "You never know unless you try," my mother said.

After coaching children in gymnastics for more than 15 years, I've seen many kids that were not naturals. They tried their best nonetheless, and accomplished some skill and felt joyful and empowered as a result. As a kid, it doesn't matter if you master a skill or are the worst in the class. Unfortunately, adults are more critical of themselves.

I was not always so active but was curious about becoming a better swimmer as an adult, having never competed as a child. So, I joined a swimming group, which led me into the sport of triathlon. If I had not experimented, I never would have discovered that swimming, running, and biking tug on my heart strings! It wasn't easy, but through hard work I learned that almost anything is possible!

What was fun for you as a child? Did you ever play sports or have any other active hobbies? If you have fun (even laugh a little), you'll get lost in the moment and possibly get swept away from the usual stresses of life.

Another lesson we can learn from youth is to find a buddy to "play with." Training partners can essentially help you with a few important things:

- Keep you accountable
- Get you in a routine

- Have fun with you
- Talking and venting (stress release)

Your buddy could be a friend or classmate from the gym, or a professional coach or personal trainer, or possibly a co-worker. All you need is someone who will be reliable. A group class with instructor and classmates also can work. Many group exercise classes, dance classes, and bootcamps have a consistent group that show up, rain or shine. Getting to know a few people will connect you and keep you accountable. Occasionally,

I organize a group of my friends to compete in a running race. Together we motivate each other, go on runs, get excited for the upcoming race, and, finally, race together. We always feel a great sense of accomplishment through a healthy bond. I've also done powerful family-bonding events with my siblings, like hiking to the summit of Mount Rainier.

An Apple a Day

Movement must happen each and every day, right? You have to get dressed, make the coffee, feed your kids, dogs, and cats. It can seem impossible. Just like brushing your teeth daily is a good idea, so is moving and sweating daily. Simple ways include cleaning your house, doing yard work, or walking your dog. But, that's the bare minimum.

Consider improving your physical health every single day to be as important as attending to your dental health. Take 30 minutes to an hour to get in a sweat session. Be creative and don't judge yourself if you're not good at it. If you're having fun, then do it daily. Imagine the consequences if you stopped brushing your teeth because of your busy day.

Momentum

The degree to which you remain fit is *your* choice. We all move around, run errands, or take care of business. We accomplish demands at the forefront of our minds, but those in the background never get done. For me, I rarely scrub the floor until my husband nags me enough to "encourage" me to get out the rubber gloves and go to work! Like me scrubbing the floor, you may have zero momentum to get in a daily sweat session. You may feel too busy putting out fires each day. Possibly, your future self can develop a motivational voice in your head to help keep your fitness and health a top priority.

Newton's first law states, "An object at rest stays at rest and an object in motion stays in motion with the same speed and in the same direction."Metaphorically, getting used to exercise is the mental equivalent of a ball rolling down a hill; if you just start your engine and add it to your daily routine, you'll get the momentum to achieve success. The hardest part is beginning, but the momentum will carry you forward and eventually become a habit.

However, it's important to remember that if you quit your routine before 12 weeks, you'll lose your momentum. This amount of time has been shown to establish the routine. Start small, and slowly build it up over time. You can even start with a 10 minute routine. Endless videos on YouTube demonstrate what to do. Just commit to yourself, and the momentum will carry you to your goal of being active. I often tell people, "Great job for showing up! That's all that really matters." Just get up, and start *moving your body*!

Outdoors is Best

What is the ideal place to move your body? Where are playgrounds located? Outside – as children well know! Research has confirmed that breathing fresh air outside will boost your mood and stimulate your body. Green exercise is physical activity in nature: parks, beaches, along rivers, through forests. It provides extremely positive benefits for mind, body and spirit that synthetic indoor locations and city streets don't provide. Green exercise[3] offers:

- More stress relief
- Clearer thinking
- Improved attention and concentration
- Enhanced mood and more happiness
- Less anxiety
- Reduced pain sensations
- Less fatigue for the same amount of physical work
- Improved quantity and quality of nighttime sleep
- Enhanced mindfulness

I have definitely experienced this first-hand! Some of my highest "runner's highs" have been jogging along California beaches. We don't all live in a sunny pleasant climate to spend much time outdoors all year round, but snow and rain can be fun too, if you have the right apparel! Try more outdoor time to get your body moving.

If It Doesn't Challenge You, It Doesn't Change You

You have an endless variety of ways to move your body, as discussed earlier: running, dancing, hiking, biking, all of which are excellent ways to achieve healthy cardiovascular benefits. As a Certified Strength and Conditioning Specialist, my approach is centered around methods that improve muscle strength and deliver cardiovascular benefits.

You can do hundreds of new, fun, and creative moves to get out of your comfort zone! I will give you a few suggestions that I have had success with, which will maximize your time and build muscle tone.

---

[3]Diana Bowler, *et al* in *BMC Public Health*

First, strength training is an excellent way to build muscle tone and to get a dynamic cardiovascular workout, too. Many people (particularly women) think they only need to get on the treadmill or elliptical machine to raise the heart rate and burn calories. This is a big mistake.

The human body needs weight bearing movements to develop a strong stable body: strong hips, balance, and even flexibility. So, consider weight bearing moves such as carrying your kids (or your groceries) up and down the stairs to achieve this goal. In fact, going up stairs is an excellent way to do some simple at-home strength movements.

Second, balance and stability moves will improve your ability to stay injury-free and protect you from falling. These little stabilizer muscles are often underused. This also includes strengthening your core and back through abdominal moves. Pilates is my preferred method, but you can be creative about firming up the midsection and experiment with yoga or any core strength class or video.

Lastly, mobility is another key component to an overall healthy body. Mobility involves relaxing moves that expand your range of motion of your joints beyond your comfort zone. Take deep breaths and let go of the tension. Mobility includes slow yoga, stretching, Pilates, myofascial release, and trigger point therapy. A relaxing massage loosens up your muscles, too!

Movement Instead of Antidepressants

We engage in activities for physical benefits and improving our appearance, but the benefits are even more important for your brain! Three hundred million people around the world experience depression, according to the World Health Organization.
Many who experience depression will never report it, therefore the number is likely higher. All of us have experienced sadness, stress, and anxiety at some point in our lives, but moving your

body and getting your blood flowing can improve your mental health.

So, to feel happier, move your body. Sweat out all that stress, raging hormones, and bad vibes! Divert your negative thoughts by playing a sport, especially outdoors in green spaces. When you're sedentary, the mind can get stuck on the same miserable thoughts.

Break the cycle by shaking it up! A good vigorous sweat session will divert your thoughts, leave you feeling relaxed, and sometimes exhausted, which may help you sleep better if you are suffering from stress-related insomnia. Finally, engaging in a new activity builds self-efficacy and subsequently, self-esteem. High self-esteem correlates with well-being, while low self-esteem is linked to mental illness.

In closing, find the inner-child who loves the playground and a big grassy field. Connect with nature in a forest, a mountainside, or a city park. Block out your inhibitions and be free to move the way you need and deserve. Be creative about simply moving however you want. By being a little adventurous, you can become light-hearted and love the simplicity of moving your body. Take care of it today, and reap the rewards tomorrow.

CHAPTER 10

Organizing for Health

By Alex Brzozowski

I don't know what my life would be like if I wasn't such a planner. With my crazy work and personal schedule, it is only by being organized that I have managed to live a balanced life, including taking care of my health.

My passion for an organized life began while I worked in law, in particular, when I was involved in distributing the assets or executing the wishes in a last will and testament.

Over and over I would witness the inability of a family to follow the desires of their loved one, due to the estate being in disorganized chaos. I resolved my commitment to develop my already strong organizational skills and share these with the world.

I also see correlation between being organized and physical well-being in my clients. If you are trying to lose weight, increase strength, eat better, or just live healthier, you may want to start looking into how you can organize everything around you.

The truth is being organized (or disorganized) affects every aspect of your life. The 13 Pillars of Health described in the Introduction can all be strengthened when you work on your organizational skills! Clutter, digital disorganization, and poor time management create overwhelm, anxiety, and stress.

These impact your mental state and trigger hormonal changes that cause weight gain as well. You may find yourself sleeping less, having cravings, eating more, getting take out, or missing your workouts because you can't stay on top of things at work or at home.

By being organized, you will experience less stress and anxiety and have peace of mind, freeing you to create and maintain the healthy lifestyle you crave. It's amazing how you can maintain a high level of energy throughout the day when everything is planned to a tee. You waste no time looking for items, and transitioning from one task to the next takes only a matter of seconds.

Organization can result by implementing the tips below. Even if you don't see yourself as a super organized person, these new habits will positively change how you feel in your day-to-day life.

Before you get started with the following step-by-step organization, it's important to assess your personal priorities. Quickly jot down how you spend your time throughout the week.

This can just be a back of the envelope calculation: if you work 50 hours and sleep 8 hours per night, you still have 40 hours per week. How do you spend them? Try to quickly make a list or, if you are inspired, a simple chart.

You may also find it useful to do the same thing with your finances: after rent and bills, how much do you spend on transportation, food, clothes, entertainment, and other categories? I realize this may be a complicated endeavor.

You can start with a guess, but consider taking the time to figure out the answer. How you spend your time and money will tell you what you are prioritizing in your life. If you want to make your health a priority, you'll need to figure out how to give it some of your time and money.

Organizing Basics

These basic organizational steps will lay the foundation for alleviating stress, the precursor to health and motivation. If you prematurely jump into "being organized" and "getting healthy" while you can't find your keys and still pay your bills late, these ongoing issues will actually derail your efforts to be healthier. Therefore, like most changes in life, start with some foundational skills and then move on, slowly improving over time.

Many books and support resources are available to assist you in determining your preferred organizing fundamentals. Once you master basic organizational skills, you can move on to more advanced ones.

Declutter. First, go through your entire home and discard any items you don't need any more. Whether you are donating to charity, selling them, or throwing them out, you need to be committed. Wondering how to clear clutter? It's about a positive mindset. If it has no use or sentimental value, let it go.

Looking at clutter or distractions not only overloads the visual cortex, but interferes with brain processes. When you're organized, you will be more efficient with less effort because you won't be over stimulated.

A simple overview of the process looks like this: First you categorize or sort your cluttered or piled items into categories. In an office this might include office supplies, paperwork, and electronics. Then you create smaller categories, such as office supplies then being divided into file folders, staples, pens, pencils, paper clips, binders, extra paper, notebooks, etc.

Categorizing helps to know what you have to make eliminating easier. For example, maybe you find out you have 10 pairs of scissors and you only need 1 or 2. If this is a new process to you, be sure to look for additional resources such as a book or hiring a professional organizer to help you get started.

Have daily routines. This is vital. Your routines can include anything from generic tasks like cleaning, to more personalized jobs such as a writing assignment. Routines reduce stress and support health and wellness.

Another noteworthy aspect about routines is that we all rely on them even if we are unaware, because "mindless habits" make our brains more efficient. The less you ponder every choice throughout the day, the more you use your brain to think, create, and enjoy. Establishing a *routine* is simply a way to become more aware and intentional with these *habits*.

Make lists. To do lists might sound a little cliché regarding organization, but they really work! Make a daily list of what you to accomplish. Checking each item off the list provides a feeling of accomplishment. Similar to creating career or business lists, you can also strategize well-being with health and wellness lists!

You should work up to a maximum of three healthy tasks per day; this is a more realistic approach and helps keep you motivated to keep going the next day. I suggest making a large list of to-dos, then breaking that down into the daily tasks so the large list isn't overwhelming. This approach leads to success!

You can also always do more than three tasks. A healthy task might be as simple as drink lemon water in the morning, eat a piece of fresh fruit, make a smoothie, go for a walk, stretch for five minutes, meditate for one minute, go to bed by a certain time, and so on.

Practice time management. As you create a new balance in your life, this may mean reintroducing daily elements previously pushed aside. Although you repeatedly told yourself you want to exercise, it slipped out of your priorities. Meal planning and healthy eating may have been hard to maintain over time.

To use your time as effectively as possible, there are two essential steps. The first trick to become more productive is to stop jumping from task to task. Cluster all similar tasks together into one block of time.

- Plan to make your phone calls back to back.
- Schedule a specific time to respond to emails (NOT as they arrive!)
- Run all errands in either one morning or afternoon, if possible.

By putting "like with like," you will actually free time in your schedule to exercise, prepare healthy food, or for any other healthy habit!

The second step is to apply this same focus to your new priority. While exercising, turn off all other distractions. Find a time when you can minimize distractions: turn off your ringer, pause your inbox, and find the time you need to focus. Turning off your phone and fully concentrating on the task at hand will manage your time effectively and encourage exercising instead of emailing.

Perhaps you already manage your time successfully regarding your job, family, or community. One of the secrets to success when it comes to making health a priority is to figure out how to organize your day to match your values (new healthy habits) with your actions. If you've had a hard time abandoning lifelong unhealthy habits, you likely have a situation in which you are valuing, for example, your productivity at work higher than your personal health and well-being. By digging a little deeper into why you are making your daily choices, you will shine light on this pattern and shift it.

Digging Deeper

Many people talk about organizing basics, but taking it to the next level for consistent results across all aspects of your life is my particular area of expertise! I love pushing my clients a little further into their thought processes around organizing so they are less likely to slip back into old habits. Taking care of the overall picture transforms other aspects of your life. The momentum just keeps going!

Identify your goals. Always identify your goal for organizing. Your primary goal drives all your decisions; this will require taking another look at your priorities and getting specific. When you know your goal, it will make it easier to keep your priorities and let go of what holds you back or makes it difficult to stay on track.

Example: Knowing you have a goal of exercising three times a week will make is easier to plan the sequence of leaving the social event early to get to bed on time so you can wake up and stick to your workout plan.

Your goal becomes your guide, and it ends up making time management decisions easier as well as other organizing decisions, such as what to keep or toss. Knowing your goal makes every decision easier.

Be proactive. There are many ways that you can be proactive in regard to organizing for health and wellness. One simple thing to do is tidy up after yourself as you go. This way you don't get overwhelmed and lose track of your designated priorities.
If things become chaotic, your new healthy goals will likely be pushed aside while you deal with the mess instead.

To keep yourself on track, you should also order your tasks from most important to least important, focusing on the top first. The most "urgent" tasks are not necessarily the most important.

Reassess how you prioritize so that yourself care, nutrition, and physical fitness remain at the top during the transition. You can look for creative ways to combine the demands on your time, such as meeting a friend for a walk instead of a drink.

Organize your digital life. One of the most essential steps to creating more free time is organizing your digital life. A few hours a week for a month will result in much more time once you know where all those photos, files, and emails are stored!

This is an overlooked but essential step to time management. We spend much of our time on computers, so when you organize your digital life, you will create more time for other important tasks, like exercising and eating healthy.

Manage your time. Time management becomes essential as you add recurring events like a workout or meal planning. Begin with planning your workouts and meal prep times well in advance. Having a solid plan keeps you on track and also allows you to anticipate and avoid distractions.

Just like scheduling appointments, schedule your workouts and make a detailed plan.

Managing time is both a basic and a more advanced organizing skill because you can continue to improve. Your schedule also benefits from all the new organizing skills by creating space for new healthy routines.

Keep your food pantry organized. This aspect of home organization gives specific attention to your kitchen and nutrition. Categorizing every item in your food pantry might seem unnecessary, but it helps you make better shopping choices.

People who are disorganized may make impulse decisions and are likely to fill up their food pantries with unhealthy foods.

Giving time to your new goal is the way you make it become a true priority. Organizing the pantry is a simple task with a clear start and finish; committing to this first task will set the precedent for the following tasks of preparing your food.

Plan your meals. It's essential to find a rhythm that keeps your healthy eating on track. For many people, the best time to do this is on a weekend. Write down the meals you intend to have in the coming week, including snacks. In addition to helping you to stick to a healthy diet, this will also save time, which can be used to relax or exercise.

Prepare for food shopping. When you shop for food unprepared, you are likely to overspend or buy food that sounds good in the moment but is likely more processed. So, if you want to maintain a healthy eating plan and minimize junk food in your refrigerator, plan your meals with a shopping list.

Fortunately, online resources can assist with meal plans and shopping lists, including the more flexible approach to meal planning in the book *Too Busy to Cook* by Alegra Loewenstein. Many convenient grocery delivery services can also help. For some people, hiring a personal chef to come to their home once a week can be a worthwhile investment. Look into your options and decide what makes most sense for you.

Seeing Results

Being organized teaches you to prepare in advance and acquire time management. This foundation ultimately becomes a lasting skill. Consistent practice will naturally lower stress levels, encourage healthier food choices, and simplify a sustained exercise program. As these take their place in your daily routine, you will find ways to expand your holistic approach to a healthy life.

With minimal time wasted and reduced stress due to better organization, your productivity will increase across the board. You will become more productive while you simultaneously create better systems at work and home; you will minimize the annoying tasks that distracted and ultimately robbed you of the time to take care of your body.

This is especially important if you are in a leadership position. New clients have often shared that they are succeeding in one aspect of life (usually career), but they are suffering in others. Yet they don't want to set this example for their peers and family.

If you are motivated to prioritize your health through exercise, nutrition, and self-care, then those around you are inspired to emulate you. From your partner or kids to friends to clients and colleagues, you become a great model for being organized and setting priorities of health and well-being.

In addition to improved health and wellness, getting organized will save time and money, freeing both of these up for a greater purpose. Organized people achieve their goals and even create the abundance to help their family or larger society. In other words, being organized can make you more charitable and allows you feel abundant through giving.

Being organized at home and in the workplace also creates time for relaxation. You finish your work on time and avoid a last-minute rush. You can rest easy because Everything will be in place. Creating time to relax will further contribute to your health, as stress is the number one reason people can't lose weight.

With clutter out of the way and your schedule complete, you will have more time to spend with your loved ones. You can sit down and enjoy a meal together, help your kids with homework, or engage in outdoor activities. Connecting with your loved ones is also an essential aspect of health.

Organization is essential to maintain a balanced and healthy life. As you look forward to achieving your wellness goals, it is important that you organize everything around you in your home or at the office. When the clutter is cleared and your digital life is in order, you will make choices that are beneficial to your health and leave ever more time for your expanding healthy habits.

CHAPTER 11

Food Mindset

By Alegra Loewenstein

This book almost didn't contain a chapter on food. Because we spend too much time thinking about food choices and weight loss, and not enough time on self-care, I thought it didn't need a chapter on food.

We spend so much effort analyzing the nutrients and calories and ratios of proteins/fats/carbs in our food. Unfortunately, that backfires. The way to lose weight permanently is to declutter our thoughts around food, to simplify. One of the secrets to lasting weight loss is to spend less time thinking about what you eat (or don't eat).

I thought teaching about other ways to look at our health would be enough. The previous chapters in this book address many ways we can release our attachment to measuring our food. The perspectives offered in this book are designed to look for internal measures of satisfaction, so we can let go of the external measures – the counting.

The previous chapters are filled with amazing insights on how to feel worthy, find the joy of movement, and learn how our traumas trap us, how to have better boundaries, to let go of stress, to really love ourselves truly and deeply, and get organized. These create the magic potion that heals us and allows us to let go of the "dieting" and the mindset of deprivation that sabotages our healthy ways.

Furthermore, I realized we need a replacement. Initially, you need to nudge the old habits out of the way to bring in the new. This approach to food will work in harmony with other forms of nourishment discussed in this book. Combining this simple approach to food with this mindset shifting approach to life will provide a "diet" to enjoy for the rest of your life.

Temptation

Imagine your daily commute. How many fast food chains do you drive by? How many convenience stores do you pass? How many opportunities to get cheap and fast food do you have? Probably more than you can count.

That is a real-life obstacle. It's really hard to keep up your healthy mindset when temptation is literally on every corner.

Worse than the temptation, we actually have people pushing junk food onto us, taking offense if we try to pass it up, or silently judging our choice. People can be weird about food! That also affects our mind and attitude and makes it harder to maintain our healthy values and goals.

So, just what is food? Michael Pollan, one of my favorite food journalists, calls 75% of what we encounter in the grocery store "food-like substances." I'm sure the fast food chains also sell food-like substances.

By this, he means that food has been so processed that, while it resembles food, it's not food in the traditional sense: Something made entirely from things that are grown or raised or harvested to be prepared in a home kitchen and eaten within a few days.

Food-like substances that surround us are terrible for our health. We must be aware how eating highly processed food or food with excessive additives changes our bodies from the hormones that drive our daily bodily functions to the microbiome of our bodies to how our DNA is expressed!!!!!

(To explain further: Our microbiome is the collection of bacteria and viruses that live in and on our bodies, and their balance is essential for our health. While our genetics are set at birth, the instructions that our genes give our body can change over time and are affected by unhealthy lifestyle choices.)

Junk food is fun to eat so the matter is complicated. For some, forbidden food makes it more desirable. I get it! It's natural to react defensively to restrictions.

Instead of viewing it as a directive, perhaps you can view it as an alternative perspective. I want to challenge you to look at this not as me "telling you something or other to do," but rather an invitation to explore and see how healthy changes make you feel.

Letting go of the idea of food as "temptation" is a radical act. Junk food can be an indulgence while still acknowledging that healthy food is delicious and nourishing. When we take away the good vs bad approach to food, food can serve us in a more holistic way.

Outside Influence

Let's take a moment to think about how advertising affects our choices. At first, we may consider ads a nuisance or a simple interruption. Perhaps we consider them a necessary evil to fund media programs we enjoy.

However, the truth is ads (and the media at large) inadvertently manipulate our emotions and affect our choices. Our complicated food choices are intricately linked to our body image.

We have received messages about our bodies our whole life. Media and advertising negatively influence our body image to promote sales.

This may sound dramatic, but pervasive influence goes right down to our family and friends, which masks it as an external force. With books dedicated to this subject, I seek to promote awareness of messaging about our bodies and food choices from outside sources that have *their* best interest in mind, not ours.

I hope you are mad right now about the undue influence of our social landscape and consequent negative self-image, designed to promote their products. Why do I hope you are mad? Because you may now be inclined to abandon your attachment to your favorite cookies, chips, crackers, pretzels, ice cream, or whatever.

Now, don't take this message wrong. You can enjoy a junky treat sometimes. I do! It's fun! But fun as a teenager or young adult is no longer aligned with my values; therefore, I don't want to indulge very often.

Emotional Eating

Of course, many of us also overeat due to emotional reasons. The previous chapters have delved into many ways to nourish and sustain yourself without relying on food. When we get to the root of the emotional triggers (I call this emotional eating detox), we can always return to the mindset that keeps us aligned with our healthy values and weight goals.

My personal journey included emotional eating, and as a health coach, I have consistently returned to the book shelf to revisit my own journey to overcome emotional eating. The evidence confirms that emotions underlying what we eat, why we eat, and when we eat are at the heart of dysfunctional eating.

People who want to lose weight generally eat too much because they have not identified and their emotional needs. Food manages their stress and meets their emotional needs. Once emotions are triggered, a whole cascade of hormones are activated, too, and make it difficult to make a healthy choice.

While this just skims the surface on this subject, I encourage you to consult books on the subject, and as well as my guided journals to explore the topic in a personal way. It takes time to accept that your emotions are behind much of your overeating. It takes time to abandon old ways and be willing to venture into scary thoughts and feelings.

The good news is action can begin with five minutes per day of contemplation and reflection. (Journals can optimize your accountability. Next, I will describe a simple new paradigm to abandon the old and welcome the new.

Stop Counting

We are trained to count, to use ideal external measures to allow outside experts to control our bodies and our choices. We must become active participants, determining the cause and effects of our actions.

There are so many ways to approach health these days. Some are the hottest trend, and others are a bit passé. I am fascinated by science and knowledge about the human body. However, when it comes to nutrition and health, the more we analyze the components and effects, the less healthy we become.

We must substitute counting calories and carbs and grams and with learn the chemistry and biology of food. It is time to reassess what our brains think, or what others have pushed onto us, and tune into our own bodies and hearts for a new approach.

You know what makes your body feel best. Before limiting carbs or fat, I challenge you to try eating whatever you want, whenever you want, but stopping when you are satisfied or not quite "full" *while also nourishing yourself in all the ways laid out in this book.*

Slowing Down

I hope you are enlightened and inspired by this book. Implementing this daily is difficult and requires that you slow down and tune into your body to honor it throughout the day so you won't need to eat to fill the void.

Abandoning negative energy makes room for healthy, nourishing activities such as choosing and preparing your food. This does not need to be complicated; it should not be determined by a running tabulation of numbers in your head.

It should involve whole food items, like potatoes and fish and cheese and chicken and vegetables and fruit that you select mindfully.

Plan your food in advance, so you don't become "desperate" to eat and consequently overeat. Healthy snacks and a few basics for a simple fresh meal are the secret.

What to Eat

If you are wondering what you should be eating, I came up with a few guidelines.

Keep it Simple. Every meal need not be fancy and complicated. People watch more TV shows about food than any time in history, yet we spend less time preparing our own food.

It is time to rediscover simply prepared foods. Quality ingredients, simply prepared are the basis of traditional foods around the world, and we owe to ourselves to rediscover that.

Buy fruits, vegetables, and ingredients. If it goes bad in a week, it's probably good for you. The effect of preservatives and the plethora of food additives found in prepared and packaged food is still largely unknown. Luckily, the list of ingredients below can help you avoid unhealthy processed foods.

Enjoy your kitchen. The kitchen must become a part of your healthy living plan. Learn to cook a few simple meals. Enjoy spending time with friends and loved ones. Take the time to enjoy real food.

Try to answer "Yes" to these items while you shop. Does your cart have fresh fruits and vegetables, including some that you will enjoy eating raw? Would you consider most of the items in your cart single ingredients? (rice, butter, salmon, almonds, etc.)

Now for the trickiest bit of all: When to say "No." No one should tell you what to eat (except a doctor who advises you based on a diagnosed medical condition).) Every bite is a choice, and it's OK to have fun eating junk once in a while.

And on the other side, it's important to develop a relationship with food where you honor your body and live your values. So, instead of making this list about being "bad" or "not allowed" – think of these as positive trigger words.

These words remind you, "This is not real food. Does my body need more nourishment today?"

The secret signal to look for is *more than ten ingredients* or any of the following words in the ingredient list:

- Artificial
- Any color #
- Preservative
- Nitrite
- Nitrate
- Hydrogenated
- Hydrolyzed
- Anything ending in "-ose" or "-ol"

What about sugar? Sugar is bad for us, but it's fun to eat! If sugar is in the first three ingredients, or if it's in the ingredients at all and it's not supposed to be sweet, then consider if an alternative would serve you better. If you are occasionally in the mood for ice cream or cake or cookies, sugar should be in the top ingredients, and you can just enjoy the sugar.

How to Eat

Eating mindfully is the secret key to success.

I know we can't always be mindful. My days are hectic, and I often have to remind myself to slow down and enjoy my food.

And sometimes I just have to wolf it down anyway because I have to run out the door, and I know it's better to eat something than not. In those cases, it's time to use the tools to help us stay on track.

Tips that are well worth implementing:

Use a small plate and small utensils. This results in smaller portion sizes (and smaller bites), naturally. Going for seconds won't necessarily be overdoing it, and taking the micro break to fill your plate may be just enough time to realize you are more satisfied than you thought. It's an opportunity to question if you really want it. If you do, go for it! If not, figure out what else could satisfy the urge.

Eat fruits and veggies first. Sometimes we just need to satisfy some of the urge to eat first, and doing it with fresh fruits and veggies is a more healthful way to do so. Keep fresh fruit and veggies on hand for the crunch time between getting home from work and actually dining.. Feel free to nosh on crudité during the interim.

Don't under eat. If you barely eat all day, and consequently use up all your energy at work, you are likely to be starving and cranky and will overcompensate at night.

Just keep in mind that tips can be limited. If you haven't addressed the mindset and identified the emotional triggers, then you will return to old habits of overeating since it is a long familiar way to deal with stress and emotions.

Overeating helped you cope with all you have to juggle in your life but it's time to find other ways to nourish, decompress, relax, sustain, and care for yourself. Taking the time to ask yourself what you actually want is a powerful tool for change. (Journaling can build this skill!)

Again, why is it worth the extra effort, even when you are in rush, to check the ingredients? Why plan meals in advance? Why double check that you have fresh food in your cart? The other chapters answer this question in detail, but I'll remind you of the basics.

Because you are worthy.

Because slowing down and finding balance is the secret to a healthy life.

Because loving your body is the only way to lose weight in a safe and sustainable way.

As long as you continue to remind yourself of these facts, and to make choices in alignment with these values, you will be on your way to a lifetime of health and happiness by allowing your body to reach its natural weight with ease!

Action Items

Just like after a successful meeting, I hope you are brimming with ideas and inspiration from the experts in this book! You've joined the story circle, and heard from successful professionals who have lost weight and found greater well-being. Instead of stopping there, process this information by completing the work pages that follow. Integrating these valuable ideas can take practice (and perhaps a quiet environment) to establish healthy life choices.

You can also find a printable copy of these action items in a worksheet format at www.alegraloewenstein.com/its-not-about-the-food.

Mindset and Weight Loss, *De'Anna Nunez*

To end emotional eating and overeating, you need to find your unconscious formula, which usually looks like this:

When I feel _____, I eat _____, and I feel better.

You Are Worthy, *Cheryll Putt*

You need to put yourself on your own priority list. If you want to get your needs met, you need to ask for them to be met.

Write down some ideas where you can ask for help, and who you can ask for it.

_____

_____

_____

_____

_____

_____

Difficulty Brings Inspiration, *Mieu Phan*

To recognize where you have an opportunity to lean into dark places, you must look for triggers.

What are things that happen in your life that make you want to disappear, run away, shut someone out, scream, punch, or pick a fight?

_____

_____

_____

_____

_____

_____

Self Care as an Act of Survival, *Trish Youse Marmo*

Find an emotion which you have not been fully confessing. Give yourself permission to acknowledge this feeling, even if just alone in your bathroom with the door locked, or in the private pages of a diary.

joy, silliness, anger, disappointment, relief, concern, fear, boredom

Add your own:

_____

_____

_____

_____

_____

Low Stress Investing, *Alegra Loewenstein*

Based on the chapter by Byron Harlan

What is your vision for the future?

_____

_____

_____

_____

_____

And what is one important goal that will help you reach that vision?

_____

_____

_____

_____

_____

_____

Emotional Well-being and Boundaries, *Melissa Rosenstock*

Set an intention in writing.

_____

_____

_____

When you honor this intention, how will it feel?

_____

_____

_____

_____

_____

Double check that the language is kind and supportive.

Weight Loss Basics, *Alegra Loewenstein*

Which will you focus on first: Getting ample sleep or ample water? Write down the obstacles that you expect to be challenges.

_____

_____

_____

Now write down a few ideas on how you can overcome these challenges or shift your mindset in order to get ample sleep or water for at least one day per week.

_____

_____

_____

_____

_____

_____

Yoga for Balance, *David Sonsara*

With eyes slightly closed, allow your mind's eye to observe the quality of your breath as you breathe deeply and feel your abdomen expand. Take a few moments to watch yourself breathe mindfully.

Next, take another few moments, while observing deeper, softer breathing from the stomach, to reflect upon your concerns. Notice what you feel and where you feel it in your body, consciously revealing the body's physical response when your mind focuses on your concerns.

Write down anything you observed.

_____

_____

_____

_____

_____

_____

Movement as Play, *Maggie Paola*

Circle three activities you'd like to try, and commit to at least one within a month!

Tennis
Ping pong / table tennis
Volleyball
Gymnastics
Basketball
Soccer
Ballet
Hiking
Swimming in a pool
Swimming in a lake
Surfing
Roller skating
Climbing a tree
Hula hoop
Line dancing
Hip hop dancing
Latin dancing
Modern dance
Dancing in your living room
Making your own obstacle course
Rock climbing (outdoors)
Rock climbing wall (indoors)
Trampoline
Yoga
Pilates

Organizing for Health, *Alex Brzozowski*

Make a healthy to do list! Make them small tasks, ideally that can be done in 15 minutes or less. Commit to checking off at least one item per week.

Food Mindset, *Alegra Loewenstein*

Write down at least three fruits and vegetables that you truly enjoy eating:

_____

_____

_____

_____

_____

_____

Then, of course, make sure you keep them stocked!

About the Authors

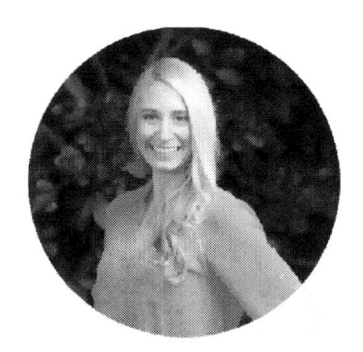

ALEX BRZOZOWSKI is a professional organizer and founder of Be Organizing. She started Be because she believes there's a better way to organize people's lives—focusing not only on the home, but specializing in digital and business organizing and productivity, including digital documents, CRM programs, photos, music, email contacts, calendar and more! Her goal is to help her clients create free time to do what they love by bringing order and efficiency into their business, digital life, and home.

www.beorganizing.com
alexb@beorganizing.com

About the Authors

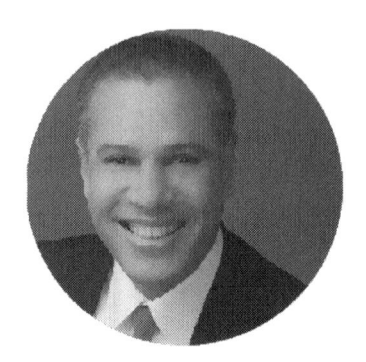

BYRON HARLAN had an award-winning career in broadcast news that spanned 30-years, before he decided to fulfill a dream he'd had for decades to become a Financial Planner. The pillars of his practice are embedded in four core concepts: compassion, truth, transparency, and independence. Byron has a bachelor's degree in political science from UCSD, a master's degree in journalism from USC, and an MBA from UC Irvine.

www.augustfinancialalliance.com
bharlan@royalaa.com

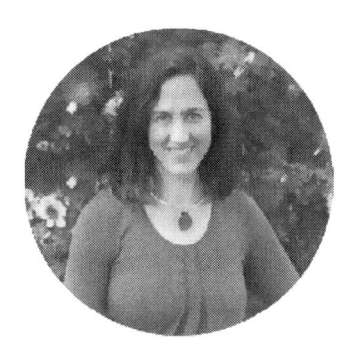

ALEGRA LOEWENSTEIN is a best-selling author, speaker, and coach on the topics of weight loss, emotional eating, and earth-based spirituality that fosters health and happiness. She is the author of two best-selling guided journals, including *Emotional Eating Detox* and *Body Wisdom Journal*. Her most recent book, *Kitchen Magic*, brings a mindset of abundance to your kitchen and health.

Alegra is an expert at helping women to lose weight in a safe and sustained way without dieting or deprivation as outlined in her recent publication *Food Journal Magic*. Alegra inspires busy, ambitious leaders to slow down, tune in to your holistic body, follow the wheel of the year, connect to your desires, cultivate your intuition, and lose weight with ease.

www.alegraloewenstein.com/freegift
alegraloewenstein@gmail.com

About the Authors

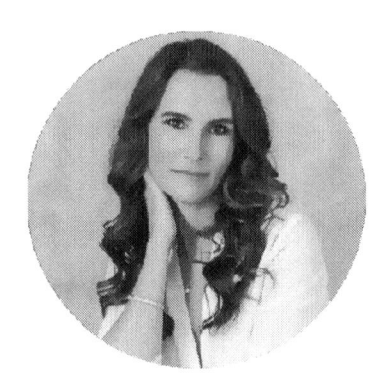

TRISH YOUSE MARMO, BSN/RN Is a National Board Certified Health & Wellness Coach, specializing in helping ambitious women over 40 lose weight and gain confidence, so they can excel in all areas of their lives. As a mom of five, and grandmother of three, her passions include her family, raising awareness for cystic fibrosis: a life-limiting, genetically inherited disease passed on to two of her children, and lifting heavy things.

As a lover of tea, ocean, and literature, she believes there's no problem that can't be solved with love, chocolate, prayer, or a good cry. She counts Robert Frost, David A. Clausen, and her grandpa, John W. Dexter, among the most influential people in her life, and she is the person she is today because of her parents. Trish currently resides in a nearly empty nest in Santa Barbara, California with her husband, Chris.

www.trishmarmo.com
trish@trishmarmo.com

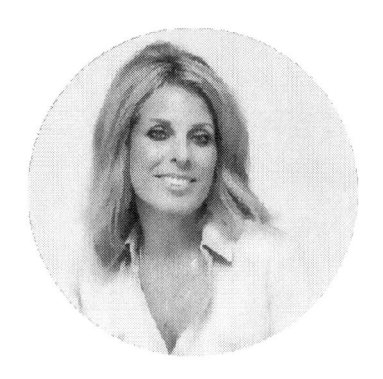

DE'ANNA NUNEZ is a Certified Hypnotherapist and author of *The F.I.T. Method*. De'Anna has created several unique health initiatives, including a program for working professionals and women across America. Ladies shed 20 to 120 pounds using hypnosis and peak performance mindset techniques.

She considers her work to be purpose driven; having felt the pain of limited confidence and indecision, she credits that very struggle as the magic that deepens her connection with her audience of learners and coaching clients. She uses hypnosis to connect people to their most vital mindset; De'Anna teaches her clients how to bypass negative thinking loops and connect to their inner reward system, to develop a deeper connection to their incentives and better manage stress and demands.

www.deannanunez.com

About the Authors

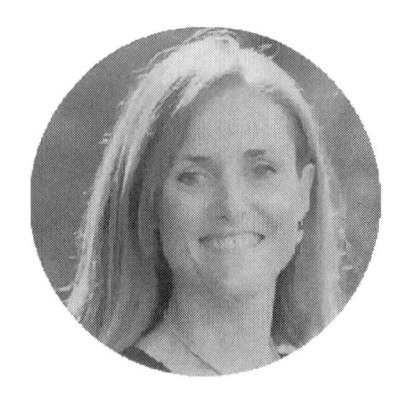

MAGGIE PAOLA is a Certified Strength and Conditioning Specialist, deeply connected to the fitness and wellness of others. Having competed in a triathlon on a national level, she's an accomplished runner, gymnast, and mountaineer.. After coaching children and adults since 2001, Maggie knows motivation is unique to each person. She takes a holistic approach, incorporating mind, body and plant-based nutrition for optimal overall health.

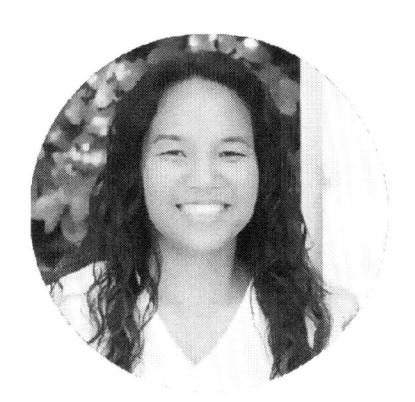

MIEU PHAN is a leadership and empowerment coach for cross-cultural integration, ex-patriots, and immigrants. She works with individuals who seek support in adjusting to a new country, in bridging the gap between cross-cultural relations, and in maximizing the potential of their expatriate employees. She opens her clients' eyes and ears to the world of their own cultural suitcase of expectations, limitations, prejudices, and baggage. Her unique perspective allows for curiosity, understanding, and sharing thus maximizing the pool of worldly views, problem-solving skills, and greater cohesion among international partners.

www.mieuphancoaching.com

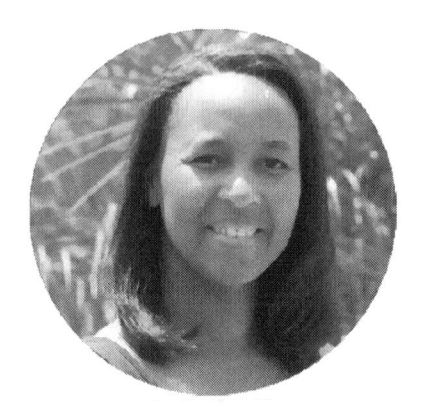

CHERYLL PUTT is a licensed therapist in private practice helping women and children heal from trauma and abuse. She is also the Single Mom Success Coach helping single mothers transform their lives to be full of empowerment, abundance, and peace. With years of clinical and personal experience, Cheryll helps her clients feel empowered to move forward into a happy and healthy life on their terms. She is passionate about elevating others through blogging, podcasting, and speaking engagements, as well as one-on-one and group coaching.

www.mommingawesomely.com
mommingawesomely@gmail.com

It's Not About the Food

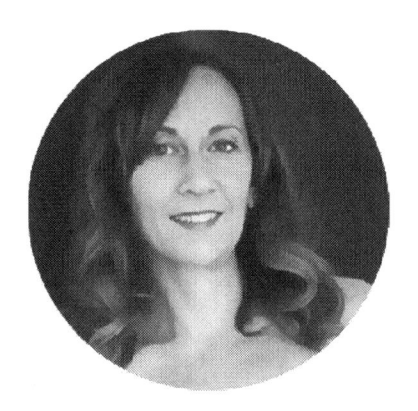

MELISSA ROSENSTOCK is a Certified International Health Coach (CIHC), specializing in helping women to create sustainable habits that optimize their health, happiness, and overall well-being. She works with women going through transitional phases of life (career change, motherhood, divorce, loss, etc.) to empower them to own their worthiness and to create a life where their own health and well-being are the top priority.

Mel gives women the tools they need to increase their energy, lose weight, feel comfortable in their skin, and create permanent healthy habits. Mel is a speaker, author, and creator of an online group program called, "Worthy & Well," empowering women to embody their worth, prioritize their health and well-being, and break free from mediocrity to create a life that nourishes their soul.

www.melissarosenstock.com
mel@melissarosenstock.com

About the Authors

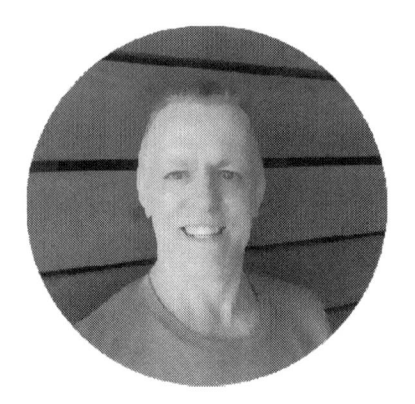

DAVID SONSARA teaches yoga, pilates, and piano. His expertise is fostering the mind-body connection, and he uses yoga and pilates to improve piano playing. His motto is, "I am still learning to listen."

www.pianofitness.com

Acknowledgements

Alegra Loewenstein

First and foremost, I want to thank my mother. She is the most balanced person I know and instilled me with a common sense approach to health, despite my tendency to go to extremes (especially in my youth).

I also want to thank my husband, for being supportive of all my ideas and endeavors and wanting me to be happy.

The contributing authors are the heart and soul of this book. Thank you, Alex, Byron, Trish, Mieu, Cheryll, Mel, David, Maggie, and De'Anna, for sharing your stories and your enthusiasm.

I also have so many wonderful and supportive family members and friends who have bought my books, written reviews, attended my events, and so much more! I appreciate your support and I am so grateful to have you in my life!!

Dad, Linda, Bob, Marla, Seren, Katie, Rosario, Laura, Jeannee, Melissa, Dan, Maryam, Chuck, Julika, Tanya, Debbie, Maren, Renae, Brittia, Heather, Sonia, April, Jenine, Cat, Mysti, and more I know must be missing!

Finally, I want to thank my improv teacher, Jacquie Lowell, for her creativity, brilliant ideas, and overall genius! This project would not be what it is without her.

Made in the USA
Columbia, SC
15 July 2019